GROUP THERAPY
IN CHILDHOOD PSYCHOSIS

*From the Child Psychiatry Unit, Department of Psychiatry,
University of North Carolina School of Medicine
Chapel Hill, North Carolina*

THE UNIVERSITY OF NORTH CAROLINA PRESS
CHAPEL HILL

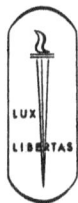

GROUP THERAPY
IN CHILDHOOD PSYCHOSIS

by

REX W. SPEERS, M. D.

and

CORNELIUS LANSING, M. D.

TO DR. LUCIE JESSNER
A Patient and Tolerant Teacher
A Devoted Friend

Foreword

Each year, for the past five years, I have visited Chapel Hill at springtime when the dogwood was in full bloom to conduct seminars in child psychiatry for residents of Duke University and the University of North Carolina. This, at least, was the official reason for the visit. I had, however, a second and more sustaining motive that made the annual journeys something of an intellectual necessity for myself. There was, in the Department of Child Psychiatry at Chapel Hill, a most unusual venture, partly therapeutic and partly investigative, relating to psychotic children. The combined interest of autism and group psychotherapy stimulated a number of my own major interests and made it seem imperative for me to remain in continued association with this project.

Once a year, therefore, I spent time in a darkened room looking in on a brightly lit, kaleidoscopic situation, sometimes of children and sometimes of parents, in various phases of communication and contact. I was a member of an invisible group that sat quietly in the dark, oriented towards the lighted window, and engaged in subdued interchanges that recalled earlier sessions of the group or drew attention to the significance of events being observed. The mirror ran almost the full length of the room thus creating a theatrical illusion of a missing fourth wall. Our observing group sat, as it were, in the penumbra of a large space and was in many ways an extension of the other group on the bright side of the one-way screen. The two groups sometimes interacted, dimly and tenuously, through chinks in the mirror and occasionally the children would visit the observers. For me, it always came as a mild shock to encounter the actors "in the flesh," making me realize how effective a thin plate of glass could be in demarcating two worlds of experience. There was no doubt, however, that the separated groups were mutually fascinated with each other and that the patients not infrequently "performed" for their audience. Small faces would be pressed against the mirrored surface, confronting us with distorted features and making our shadowy selves self-conscious at being observed in our turn.

I have often thought that in my visits to Chapel Hill, I was involved in observing the growth and development of two different group organizations, the treating and the treated. Both groups showed considerable changes over this period of time. The treating group gained in confidence with respect to understanding its own reactions and those of the patients, whilst in the treated group, there was an increasing emergence of genuine, spontaneous, personal and interpersonal feelings. I was in a good position in my role as annual visitor to appreciate the dramatic transformations that occurred. Originally, I had predicted that therapeutic developments might be slow and that therapists might find it difficult to obtain even a small quota of treatment satisfactions from this type of patient. I also predicted that the treating group, for this reason, might lose interest and find justifications for terminating the therapeutic contract. I was wrong on both counts. Not only were the changes striking with each successive year, but the group of therapists evolved into a dedicated, enthusiastic team whose daily lives were so much saturated with the group experience that they even took it home to their families and, no doubt, had dreams indicating involvement in depth. (I always recall the wonderful dream I had of my first non-speaking psychotic child with whom I conducted an elaborate dream conversation a few months after I had started intensive treatment with him.)

The reason for this degree of investment in time and interest is not too easy to understand. The challenge of unresponsiveness is certainly great, but the discomforts of uncontrolled group behavior are not to be underestimated. The impact of primitive fantasy, incomprehensible and disturbing, is as likely to repel as to attract the therapist. The weak nature of the interpersonal ties and the poverty of genuine group formations are not conducive to interesting process developments or to the unfolding of interlocking dynamic mechanisms. What then holds the therapists and patients together over the years? From my own second-hand experience of the situation, I was left with the feeling that a major contributing factor lay in the metamorphosis that led gradually, and almost inevitably, to the emergence of a communicative, conscious, co-operative self out of something impersonal and anonymous. It is tantamount to the creation of a human child, and it is therefore not too surprising that these department offspring stimulate strong parental responses in their caretakers.

From the visitor's eye view, the growth of identity from increasing individuation was more salient than for the resident community. It seemed, quite suddenly, one springtime, that the children were no longer specimens of morbidity but people, and people with recognizible idiosyncracies. As I previously indicated, the rate of change came as a real surprise and led me to wonder to what extent this was related to the technique involved or to the enthusiasm and persistence of the treating group. Was it simply a case of pioneering zest or could one reasonably expect the results to be replicated by any other group of workers adhering to the same plan of treatment? If I had not been in the position to inquire more closely into the attitudes and motives of the team and to be informed of the course of treatment in detail, I might have subscribed to the "Western Electric" hypothesis. Being acquainted, however, with the vicissitudes of the group histories, the ups and downs and the progressions and retrogressions, the rethinking of theoretical and practical issues at moments of impasse, I was led to the conclusion that group techniques, tried by the fire of experience, were being applied with increasing subtlety and clear-mindedness and that a therapeutic regime, rooted in rational considerations, was the natural outcome. As in all therapeutic undertakings, trial and error were certainly at work, but as time went on, the errors were less in evidence although the therapists remained as flexible and as open-minded to possible treatment maneuvers as ever.

Previous to this, I had not myself experienced a therapeutic program of similar complexity, and I must confess it often left me feeling very bewildered. The first year of the project, my role had been that of an expert with special knowledge both of autistic children and group processes. I found that when the two were put together, my *expertise* sounded less assured, and as the years went on, I became increasingly a student, gratefully learning from an extraordinary undertaking. My annual "busman's holiday" procured me a privileged ringside seat in what the authors referred to as a "three-ring circus," at the same time absolving me from any responsibility for what was being done. At times, I felt guilty at having so easily available the fruits of the hard therapeutic work that continued week in and week out throughout the year. It is from this vantage point that I would like to comment on some of the phenomena presented to my attention.

An immediate feature that impressed this observer was the multiple shades of childhood psychosis that revealed themselves in this group interactional setting. In the course of ordinary clinical work, one becomes accustomed to thinking of pathological states in terms of a simple, static conglomeration of symptoms. Here one was able to note how dynamic, variable, and shifting was the clinical picture. Having also been in the habit of loosely acquainting the psychotic with the archaic, I was surprised to observe the "high level" psychopathology that made its appearance in the group setting, often in very dramatic form. Castration anxieties, for example, would sometimes appear on catastrophic occasions when the primitive egos of the children were struggling with a complex of anxieties stemming from every stage of development, the whole being acted out in a concrete and literal manner. It came as a relief to witness this familiar "high level" psychopathology among the unknown terrors that hinted at annihilation, fragmentation, disorganization, and loss of all personal identity.

Another somewhat unexpected discovery had its origin in the system of parallel group sessions of children, mothers, and fathers that provided a rich opportunity for correlating responses within families. The same unconscious ideas appeared to dominate each member of the family, so that children could almost be "blindly" matched with their fathers and mothers on the basis of such productions. This was another unexpected "high level" response, since I had not expected to find such a close correspondence in fantasy content between parent and psychotic child. It would seem that the systems of unconscious communication operate as potently as they do in normal and neurotic parent and child transactions.

I would like to say a word here about the therapeutic uses made of the arrangements in the therapy room. The one-way mirror became an invaluable adjunct to the therapeutic process. The children used it to learn about themselves, their body parts and the way in which affects obtained facial expression. This was especially important in the early stages of the group when they were unable to look directly either at themselves or at others. The mirror provided a less threatening extension of the group world in which people and events could be observed obliquely. A certain amount of experimentation with reactions was possible in this mirror world before it was tried out in the real environment. The mirror was also a help in controlling panic, although it is possible that at times it contributed to group panic as a result of reflecting the chaos and confusion that took possession of the group from time to time. For members of the group, with an eye on the mirror world, it would seem almost as if twice as much of everything was taking place. Under conditions of the small room, the mirror, and the group of therapists and children, any element of disorganization could make the therapeutic environment seem very crowded. I sometimes felt, in an attempt to empathize with the psychotic child, that it must be really difficult to remain autistic under such circumstances.

The mirror reflections must have offered the therapists a cue to further adventures in technique. With much ingenuity, they began to reflect in their own comments the affects and behavior of the children. At an early stage, when verbal output in the group was low, these verbal reflections made a singular contribution to group life, making it seem as if a significant level of communication was being maintained. The reflections also conduced to the growing awareness in the child of his own activities and feelings as distinct from the activities and feelings of others.

The inclusion of a toilet in the therapeutic environment demonstrated once again how a simple physical facility could become a cornerstone in the treatment situation, especially when wisely used by the therapeutic team as a means of differentiation and individuation. The acts of urination and defecation thus became an essential part of group life when various aggressive and libidinal possibilities were tested out. The separation of the person from his feces simulated on a different plane the separation of the self from the non-self, and it was repeatedly demonstrated to the group that the self was able to endure even when excreta made their mysterious disappearance into an unknown, underground world. It was around these inchoate pregenital preoccupations that the counter-transference reactions of the therapists began to focus, and it raised questions as to what degree of permissiveness was therapeutically permissible. The primitive excitements occasioned by the display of primitive materials and primitive functions resulted in much group wildness that must have been difficult for the therapists to live through and work with. True, however, to their flexible attitude to trial and error, they experimented with various possibilities offering sublimations, suppressions, structures, and alternate satisfactions in an attempt to keep it under therapeutic control. A great deal of group discussion went on among the therapists and, as a result, they decided to work with the primitive impulses until the group was able to exercise its own controls and exorcize its own devils. My experience with psychotic children in the group situation has convinced me that some work has to be done by the primitive ego before cosmos can proceed out of chaos. World order cannot be decreed for this type of child; it has to be achieved through gradual and painful steps.

I cannot bring this foreword to a close without recounting an interesting incident that took place in the children's group recently. It is illustrative of the way in which the group setting helps to clarify an individual piece of psychopathology. One of the children developed a strong attachment for a stuffed rabbit. In his own development, the rabbit began to play a multitude of roles and to fulfill a variety of needs. At an early stage, it was very much a psychotic fetishistic object regarded animistically by the child. Later, it had many of the properties of a "transitional" object and still later a treasured object on the way to becoming a play thing. At the time of the incident, it was still highly cathected so that boy and rabbit were often inseparable, and boy was highly protective and possessive about rabbit. The group became interested and involved in the relationship, especially as the boy frequently provoked them to acts of intervention. On an occasion, I was watching the group in the playground from an upstairs window. The boy was blatantly tempting the group to dare to harm his rabbit and soon had another child engrossed in the desire for taking possession of the stuffed animal. He made several attempts to do so but was defeated on each occasion by the owner who eventually placed the rabbit apparently out of reach on a fence. Within seconds, the thief had leaped on it and gained possession, holding it closely within his arms. It was at this point that a look of intense disappointment showed on his face. The magic that had been built up over the months through its use as a fetishistic and transitional object could clearly not be transferred from the owner. It was just a stuffed rabbit and nothing more and he relinquished possession immediately without a struggle. The internalized representation of the external object had not been built up in the second boy and he had found himself with an uncathected object.

I think that at the end of this account, readers will be prepared to agree with the authors that group psychotherapy of psychotic children is not only feasible and practical but even desirable, since the symbiosis the child makes with the group ego gives it a chance to carry through its work of emancipation from the unhealthy tie to the mother. The exposure to group is not devoid of initial panic and crisis, but when the support is as complete as that offered in this therapeutic investigation, the child is clearly able to live through it and learn through it.

What is especially gratifying to me is that the small germ of an idea offered many years ago should have grown and taken shape in this impressive way. What began as a suggestion for group psychotherapy with psychotic children was extended into a group organization for families with a psychotic child and has culminated, so it seems to me, in a therapeutic group culture that looks enduring. It is my belief that the group approach to the traditional problems of psychopathology may bring about new facets of understanding, built into a composite picture through joint investigations conducted by individual and group methods.

E. James Anthony, M.D.
St. Louis
November, 1964

Acknowledgments

This project is a joint effort of the following sections of the Department of Psychiatry, North Carolina Memorial Hospital: Child Psychiatry, Psychology, Social Service, Nursing, Occupational Therapy, and Recreation.

Participants have included: Brenda Ball, A. John Bambara, Barbara J. Booth, Robert R. Byrd, Dennis D. Carmichael, Frances C. Cleary, Barbara H. Cleaveland, Andrew J. Courts, June F. Crews, Betty L. Davis, Olene H. Davis, Leah E. Fitch, Dorothy A. Forrester, Jeanne D. Harbour, Gene A. Hayes, Robert B. Hughes, Cornelius Lansing, Claudeline P. Lewis, Herman P. Lineberger, Sue Luter, Nancy Gordon McGirt, Barbara J. Maxwell, Alton R. Mayberry, R. Ramsey Mellette, Dale C. Morter, Richard C. Parker, Janet L. Reece, Maria P. Reyes, Hugh W. Ridlehuber, Ruth Faison Shaw, Angela J. Everette Smith, Rex W. Speers, Lillian Alice Spencer, Cynthia E. Swisher, Lon E. Ussery, and Jean T. Watts.

Dorothea Scott Whitten, Rosa Lee R. Golub, and Marsha L. Nunn of the Sociology Department observed the sessions and rendered valuable aid in understanding group formation and interaction. Special education teachers were Catherine C. Merritt and Margaret D. Lansing.

Ruth Faison Shaw conducted finger painting classes for a group of mothers.

A number of visiting psychiatrists observed therapy sessions and contributed important clues to the understanding of the over-all dynamic problems and specific items of enigmatic behavior. These included Drs. E. J. Anthony, George Gardner, Haim Ginott, Kenneth Gordon, Margaret Mahler, Richard Masland, and James T. Proctor.

This project was supported in part by USPHS NIMH Grants #5 R11-MH-1205-02 and 5 R11-MH-1206-02.

Contents

GROUP THERAPY
IN CHILDHOOD PSYCHOSIS

I · Introduction

The purpose of this monograph is to report a four-year study of the feasibility and effectiveness of group therapy in the treatment of young psychotic children and of the collateral group therapy of their parents.

In the spring of 1960, four psychotic children, $3\frac{1}{2}$ to $4\frac{1}{2}$ years old, were referred to our clinic for treatment, which we could not provide in the traditional way because of a shortage of individual therapists. At the same time, personal contact with E. J. Anthony [1] of St. Louis gave rise to an idea for a novel approach to the problem—group therapy. Mahler and Furer's [2] work correctly implies that therapy of the symbiotic psychotic child can take place only in the framework of a symbiotic relationship, which is presumably restricted to a one-to-one relationship with the therapist. In his group therapy work with older children, Anthony postulated the formation of a "group ego," which provides support to the defective egos of the individual patients. He suggested that for young psy-

1. S. H. Foulkes and E. J. Anthony (1957), *Group Psychotherapy: The Psychoanalytic Approach* (Baltimore, Penguin Books).
2. M. S. Mahler and M. Furer (1960), Observations on research regarding the "symbiotic syndrome" of infantile psychosis, *Psychoanalytic Quarterly*, 29:317–327.

chotic children the "therapeutic symbiosis" necessary for treatment could be similarly provided by a "group ego" developed in group therapy. Accordingly, we decided to form a therapeutic group from the four psychotic children on our treatment waiting list.

THE CHILDREN

The four youngsters had been referred to our center from several psychiatric facilities, where they had been diagnosed "childhood psychosis with autistic features." Re-evaluation confirmed the diagnosis in each instance. A fifth child joined the group five months later. The diagnostic criteria were those outlined by Mahler, Furer, and Settlage: [3] "(1) alienation, or withdrawal from reality, and (2) severe disturbances in the individual child's feeling of self-identity." The children's most prominent behavioral symptoms were as follows:

1) Language defects—total absence of speech in one child; incomprehensible gibberish in two; stereotyped phrases devoid of communicative content in one. One had infantile speech with misuse of pronouns (example: "You want a cookie," rather than "I want a cookie").

2) All but one child lacked bowel and bladder control.

3) All the children had severe sleeping and eating disturbances.

4) All showed unusual fascination with television commercials and things which turned or could be twirled.

5) All showed various forms of repetitive stereotyped behavior, and complete withdrawal from

3. M. S. Mahler, M. Furer, and C. F. Settlage (1959), Severe emotional disturbances in childhood, in S. Arieti (ed.) *American Handbook of Psychiatry* (New York, Basic Books) Vol. 1, pp. 816–839.

other human beings, to such an extent that parents felt they could not make contact or communicate with the children, and wondered if they might be deaf.

6) All had severe tantrums, with indiscriminate destruction of inanimate objects and alarming self-destructive behavior such as head-banging and biting of the hand and arm.

7) Every child had at one time exhibited unusual sensitivity to light, touch or sound.[4]

Four of the children were thought to have symbiotic psychosis [5] while the fifth (Tina) suffered from primary infantile autism (in the sense of Kanner).[6] In each of the former there had been a definite point in time at which regressive behavior had begun: 3½ years with Bob, following a sudden trauma, and between 12 and 15 months with Mike, Walter, and Annaletta, after prolonged and severe conflict in the mother-child relationship.

Pediatric and neurological examinations, including electroencephalograms and endocrinological studies, revealed no significant pathology. Although the neurological findings are normal, several observers have had an unconfirmed impression of diffuse, mild brain damage in one child; a second child has the appearance of mental deficiency. There was no history of significant birth trauma in any of the children; one had been delivered by cesarean section because of placenta previa, but post-partum examination of the child was normal.

Psychological tests supported the impression of psychosis, but formal testing of intelligence was not possible.

4. P. Bergman and S. K. Escalona (1949), Unusual sensitivities in very young children, *Psychoanalytic Study of the Child,* 3–4:333–352.

5. M. S. Mahler (1952), On child psychosis and schizophrenia: Autistic and symbiotic infantile psychoses, *Psychoanalytic Study of the Child,* 7:286–305.

6. L. Kanner (1949), Problems of nosology and psychodynamics of early infantile autism, *American Journal of Orthopsychiatry,* 19:416–426.

There is much mental illness to be found in the close relatives of these children. Bob's father suffered three episodes of severe depression, requiring 2-3 months' hospitalization each time; his mother had a moderately severe post-partum depression, and had a near-psychotic reaction during therapy. Annaletta's mother is an ambulatory schizophrenic. Tina's mother suffered an acute psychotic episode (not requiring hospitalization) during therapy. Mike's paternal great-aunt had a psychotic episode followed by suicide. There is no history of psychosis in Walter's family, although his father has severe obsessive-compulsive symptoms. There is evidence of serious character disorder and neurotic marital interaction in nearly all the grandparents.

The outstanding personality feature of the mothers is their marked immaturity and narcissism, exemplified by their profound rage over frustration of their dependency wishes. The fathers also have serious dependency conflicts, but handle frustration by physical and emotional withdrawal from their wives, to avoid perception or expression of angry feelings. The mothers quickly formed a coherent therapy group, but in the fathers' group physical absence was frequent and group formation difficult to obtain.

Group therapy with these children began in May, 1960, and is continuing. By the end of four years, the children had been seen twice weekly for a total of 828 hours. On Tuesdays the children were seen for 3 hours of group therapy, and the mothers for $1\frac{1}{2}$ hours of group analytic therapy. On Fridays the children were seen for another session of $1\frac{1}{2}$ hours. Group therapy for the fathers began in the ninth month of the program, and was held during the Friday children's sessions. The schedule was set up this way because of the rigors of travel: three of the families lived between 50 and 170 miles from Chapel Hill. In addition to the authors and psychiatric residents, co-therapists have been drawn from volunteers from many disciplines, including nursing, psychology, occupational therapy, and recreational therapy, as well as non-professional personnel such as clinic secretaries. During the fourth year of the program a formal teaching and crafts program occupied the major portion of each session.

As an integral part of the program, each family hired a colored "mammy" who was to be in the home 8 hours a day, 5 days a week, to relieve the mother of responsibility for the physical care of the sick child as much as possible. She was instructed to play with the child at whatever level he wished and to gratify as many of his wishes as possible. We had hoped the "mammy" would provide the child with an alternative to the constant anxiety-provoking interaction with the mother. In practice, however, we discovered that the mothers' jealously prevented them from hiring the desired type of "mammy." In most cases a maid was hired to perform the household duties, while the mother continued her intense interaction with the child. In those instances where an adequate "mammy" was hired, the tensions resulted in her being dismissed within a short period of time. The mothers withheld information about the "mammy," and it was only when the social scientist made home visits that the inadequacy of the hired maid was discovered. However, undoubtedly the hired maid did interact somewhat with the child.

In an effort to obtain more verbalization of fantasy, each child was seen individually by an occupational therapist, 45 minutes each week, from the tenth month of therapy. At the same time, the mothers began attending a finger-painting class, as a group, once a week.

When the fifth child was added to the group, her mother was seen in weekly individual therapy by a psychiatric resident.

After 13 months of therapy, the original group of children had progressed to the point where group formation was a reality and various degrees of separation-individuation had occurred: all were free from panic reactions; all were talking; all were toilet trained and sleeping and eating without difficulty, and therapy was proceeding nicely. At that point four additional children were added. Of these, two had symbiotic psychosis with autistic features, one was a borderline psychotic, and the fourth a mentally defective child with psychosis. This last child was withdrawn by the mother after four months of therapy in spite of obvious improvement. A second child from the added group was removed after less than a year of therapy when the family moved to another state. During the fourth year of therapy, two more children (girls) were added to the group.

In the next chapter we will present case histories of the original five children, including sketches of the parents' family backgrounds, marital interaction prior to the birth of the child, and a description of the family's life up to the beginning of treatment. This will be followed by description of the activities of the children's therapy group and of certain events which influenced our hypotheses about the nature of childhood psychosis. Next we will present interactions in the mothers' and fathers' therapy groups and the material from which we deduced hypotheses concerning the family dynamics of childhood psychosis, which will then be discussed in detail. In the final chapters we will outline events in the later phases of the children's therapy.

II · The Children

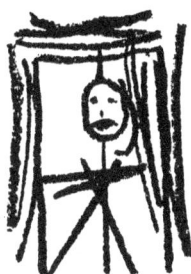

WALTER W.

Walter W. (born 11-18-56, age 3½ at start of therapy) was the unwanted child of a 29-year-old obsessive-compulsive minister and his 26-year-old emotionally immature wife. A brother was born when Walter was 27 months old. At three years of age, Walter was not talking, not relating to other children, not toilet trained, and would spend the entire day twirling objects, completely absorbed in himself and unresponsive to commands or other verbal communications.

Walter's Mother

Walter's mother was the fourth of five girls, born when her father, a minister, was 55, and her mother, a school teacher, was 38. The eldest child was seven years older than Mrs. W. (Kay), and the second and third children died in early infancy, prior to Kay's birth. Her mother was greatly concerned that Kay too might die in infancy and moved from the home to an apartment next to a hospital so as to be near help should the infant become ill. Mother and Kay lived in this apartment for one month and then returned to the family home. Mrs. W. recalls being lectured to about staying in the yard, not getting off the porch, not playing in the street, and how a neighbor boy was hired to chase her home with threatening gestures should she disobey. One of her earliest memories was of deliberately allowing a door to slam on her fingers. At two years of age her older sister became ill, and mother moved out of the house for eight months to devote herself exclusively to the care of this sick child. A series of cats, which Kay felt to be her sole possessions, were taken from her, which made her feel lonely and bitter toward her parents. She slept with her father until age ten and recalls feeling that the mother intruded upon this relationship. She sums up her early relationship with her mother as one in which she could completely control her mother but wished mother would make her do things rather than giving in to her all the time. When Kay was four years old her younger sister was born, and she vividly recalls the intense hatred and jealously she felt toward her and how this continued into adult life. Her early life seemed beset with contradictions and chaos: a "fire-and-brimstone" preacher for a father, and a mother incapable of dealing with her children. Her peer group relationship was characterized by a feeling of being better than all the other children, but she also had intense feelings of inadequacy. Her first close "chum" relationship began in college, although there were earlier crushes on female school teachers. She met her husband during the college years, and although he fitted perfectly her "checklist for suitable mates," she was aware of their inability to "let themselves go" emotionally. Sexual interests became a problem after eighteen months of steady dating, and marriage was the only acceptable solution. The conception of Walter during the fifth month of marriage was unplanned and undesired. The pregnancy was uncomplicated, but delivery occurred only after 27 hours of hard labor. She expressed great disappointment that Walter looked like his father's mother, toward whom she felt jealously and hatred. Her thoughts about the baby were: "In his perfection, my imperfections will leave." She described tremendous uncertainty about the care of this child—she was unsure whether to pick him up, lay him down, let him sleep, wake him up, feed him, or play with him. She constantly wished for someone to advise her. Difficulties in her husband's parish resulted in considerable marital strife. A move to an even less desirable parish accentuated this, but here she did participate in much of the church activity. She later recognized this as a way of getting away from her anxieties over Walter's care. When Walter was 18 months old she conceived again, and during the seventh month of pregnancy she developed kidney stones. For the next four months she was in and out of the hospital and had surgery two months post-partum. Mrs. W. had a brief contact with psychotherapy during her junior year in college, intensive psychotherapy for a year prior to her marriage and again shortly after Walter's birth. Although she feels her psychotherapy accomplished a good deal, she still feels inferior, incompetent, distraught, and quite unable to cope with the problems of her marriage, and indecisive about discipline and other matters relating to the children.

Walter's Father

Walter's father was the middle of three children (he has two

sisters) born to a mother twenty years younger than her husband. The mother was the dominant person in a strife-torn
household who insisted upon absolute submission to her will.
Mr. W. (Walt) decided early to dedicate himself to a life of
"doing good for others." He worked his way through school,
denying himself most worldly pleasures, and struggled
mightily over the question of whether to marry or to be free
to give his all to humanity. Obsessive concern over words
containing four letters led to compulsivity in his writings and
sermons. His early resolve never to indulge in heated verbal
interchange has caused him to assume an aloof attitude in his
relationship with his wife and children. Under the aegis of
liberal protestantism, he is indulgent towards the behavior and
attitudes of others but demands strict conformity of himself
as though he was destined, like Christ, to suffer for the sins
of all mankind.

Developmental History

Although the pregnancy was uncomplicated, Walter's mother
suffered great anxiety and fears throughout. She was informed
that her inability to relax caused the prolonged labor. Walter
weighed 7 pounds, 11 ounces at birth; he breathed and cried
spontaneously and the nurses said that he slept most of the
time and cried less than the other babies in the nursery. This
pleased his mother, for she dreaded the thought of a crying
baby. He was breast fed for nine months, with supplemental
bottle feedings. He was alert in the hospital, looking about
the room, but would fall asleep immediately after nursing.

In her autobiography (requested of all the parents by the
therapist) mother wrote: "Walt and I were afraid that we
would handle him wrongly, so we calculated everything we
did for him and with him. We wanted everything to be just
right. We felt that environment determined one's orientation
to life, and we wanted our baby to be perfect." She did not

want to "spoil" him, so that even though she had urges to play with him, she dutifully put him back to bed after feedings. She was very concerned about his being too dependent on her, and decided to ignore most of his crying, all of his sneezing, and later his falls when he attempted to walk. She recalls that when she was angry or preoccupied with her own thoughts, she would not utter a sound to the baby while bathing, dressing, or diapering him. He exhibited fears of falling while she bathed him and violently resisted her washing out his eyes and mouth with boric solution and washing his penis and scrotum. He enjoyed being cuddled and was ecstatic when swung between mother's legs. People complimented mother on having the calmest and happiest baby they had ever seen. Mother, however, felt that he *should* be happy, inasmuch as she did everything for him and gave him everything he wanted; he therefore had "no reason to cry."

Between eight and twelve months of age, mother left him in the playpen for hours at a time while she busied herself in other parts of the house. He would rock the pen violently to attract her attention and would force her to take him out. During this period mother and father slept upstairs while Walter slept downstairs. Mother guiltily admits that he cried almost every morning, and that she did not know how long he had been crying before she heard him. To forestall his impatience, she put toys in his bed for him to amuse himself with before she awakened. She describes his reaching out to her, crying for her, and saying "mama" when she entered the room. She early put a fuzzy animal in his crib, which he retained during the first year of therapy. At nine months of age, she noted in her baby book that he was making noises by uttering "strings of syllables." At this time he was able to drink from a cup, but because it was easier for her, mother preferred to give him the bottle and did not bother with the cup. Even though he early tried to feed himself, she would not permit this, thinking him to be incapable. In short, it appears that Walter made numerous attempts to mature but was repeatedly forced to remain infantile.

Following brief hospitalization for an upper respiratory infection at 14½ months, Walter's feeding patterns regressed, and he showed progressive signs of withdrawal. Mother accompanied him to the hospital, and when he returned home he would eat nothing but pureed foods, and only if spoon-fed by his mother. He continued to sleep much of the time—12 hours at night and 3 to 4 hours in naps. He played by himself at all times, repetitively taking a toy apart and putting it together again, and did not seem to care whether mother was present or not. She decided he needed some other children to play with but he completely ignored those she provided.

When Walter was 18 months old his mother conceived again, and during the latter part of pregnancy, she had serious difficulty with kidney stones. While she was hospitalized for renal colic, delivery, and finally surgery, father took over Walter's care and readily fell into the pattern of treating him just as mother had done. When mother returned, Walter paid little attention to her. Since then, she has noted whenever she returns from being away from Walter, he hits her in the stomach. The advent of Tim proved that Walter had some awareness of others, for he displayed overt aggression toward his brother. Mother describes many times when she entered the room and found Walter in Tim's crib, trying to stamp on the baby's head with his feet. It never occurred to her to remove Tim's crib to an inaccessible place. About this time, mother and Walter developed an exciting game. Walter would dash wildly to the room where mother was working. She would shout, "Here he comes!" and greet him with joyful expressions. He would then turn and run into another room, and mother would shout, "There he goes!" This was repeated many times throughout the day.

As Walter neared three years of age, mother became increasingly aware that something was wrong: "He *could* drink from a cup; I had seen him pick up a bucket of water from his pool and drink it. But *why* didn't he drink at the table? He *could* hear and talk, for he would parrot words to me. But *why* didn't he go on talking? He was interested in watching the commode flush. But *why* wouldn't he sit on the commode? He *would* hum songs to himself and pick out tunes from the phonograph. But *why* wouldn't he tell us what he wanted? He would sit for hours and twirl *objects* but would not play with *us* nor pay *any* attention to us."

Initial Contact with Walter

In the diagnostic interview with Walter, he showed no re-action to being separated from either parent and paid no atten-tion to them when they said goodbye. He also showed no reaction to the examiner, nor to the room itself. He noted the toys and perfunctorily inspected them. He ultimately found a rubber dart which he pressed against the wall and seemed in-terested in the noise it made when he pulled it off. He then looked at the psychiatrist for the first time. He spent the re-mainder of the time sticking the dart on the wall and pulling it off. He appeared interested when the psychiatrist imitated the sound with his tongue. He did not respond to the spoken voice and showed no interest in shooting the dart from the gun which the examiner offered. When the psychiatrist built a pile of blocks, Walter built a similar pile but his attention was devoted to making certain that all the blocks had the letters on top. When it was suggested that he might like to knock down the blocks, Walter paid no attention, but as he was about to leave, managed to kick the blocks over with a show of pleasure. In an interview with the psychologist, Walter played with the form board and refused to give it up and would not respond to other test objects placed before him. He did exhibit skill when using it, and when it was taken from him, he had a tantrum. He became interested in the rod to the filing cabinet, and after watching the examiner remove it one time, was able to duplicate this action with a pleased expression. He did not respond to commands or requests and displayed no inclination to please either the psychologist or his parents. In a second interview he was even less responsive and would only spin a toy during the entire hour.

Course in Group Therapy

During the first six sessions, Walter's behavior was like that of a child with primary autism. He entered the room, put his thumb in his mouth, looked down at the floor, and remained oblivious to everyone in the room. He made no move toward his mother when she left or when she returned. He eventually picked up a stuffed animal from the floor, found his way to a corner where he sat, sucked his thumb, and rubbed the toy against his nose. He refused all contact with adults and children, and if a child bumped into him, he merely moved away. He refused cookies and milk by turning his back. At times he removed a knob from the phonograph and sat twirling it or any other round object he could find. Often he stood by the phonograph for the entire period, watching the record spin. Toward the end of the sixth session, he took note of the mirror which covered one wall of the room. He did not look at his own reflection, but used the mirror to observe the other children. During the seventh session he first looked at the other children in the mirror, then at himself. He then went completely around the room sucking his left thumb, with his right thumb on his nose and the right forefinger extended so as to touch the wall. He then went to various sections of the room and seemed to be delineating the area with thumb in mouth and index finger extended. He similarly explored the

phonograph and other objects in the room. In the same manner, he traced the outline of his image in the mirror. At this
point he dared to turn around and peep directly at the other
children, at first furtively, with frequent glances back into the
mirror, but ultimately looking at the children directly without
utilizing the mirror.

In the following sessions he developed a new behavior pattern in which he entered the room as though excited, ran to the
toy box, and threw everything in it up to the ceiling. He then
looked at the male therapist, laughing and seemingly inviting him to chase him. He was chased and caught. He laughed
and giggled with obvious pleasure and repeated the sequence
over and over. He permitted no one to pick him up, nor would
he participate in any other game or activity. He ultimately
went after the cookies, devouring all he could get his hands
on, but declined the milk by crying, making an angry sound,
and turning away. When his mother returned to get him, he
struck out at her, hitting her in the abdomen. His behavior
toward the other children became more aggressive, and soon he
was hitting, kicking, pulling, and biting them. When we
attempted to restrain him, he became panicky, cried, tried to
wriggle away, and kicked and hit at the restraining person.
When by himself, he cringed when an adult approached him.
The game of throwing toys continued, and we learned that
he also did this a great deal at home; it seemed as if he
were symbolically "throwing away" the other children, as he
wished to "throw away" his brother. When Annaletta entered
the group, she became a particular target of his aggression.
Finally, the other children ganged up on him and retaliated en
masse for his aggressive behavior. As this was repeated several
times, his own aggression became less indiscriminate and was
confined to situations in which property rights and desires were
involved. He gradually participated in more of the group
games and soon was an active leader in playing ring-around-

a-rosy, run and chase, clapping hands to tunes, and catching the ball.

Interaction of Walter W. Family

Significant pathological interactions and identifications exist in Walter W.'s family: The overindulged, infantilized mother; the masochistic, "saintly" father; the infantile, hedonistic child. Mrs. W. presented herself as a helpless child, totally incapable of coping with the demands of her environment. She identified with Walter, treating him according to her own neurotic wish to be babied. Her fantasy of being a "little princess" appeared in many forms, and when her "royal" wishes were frustrated, the intensity of her rage was remarkable. When the father was unable to gratify his wife's demands she responded with tremendous rage against him, but because of his need to avoid the emotion of anger, he withdrew (emotionally and/or physically) from the situation and assumed an aloof attitude. He was aware that this withdrawal enhanced his wife's rage, but he steadfastly refused to become involved in "mundane emotions." Mrs. W.'s rage was then directed toward the child.

The symbiotic quality of the mother-child relationship was displayed in Walter's behavior in therapy: he insisted that the female worker assist him in all tasks, and in return he helped her as though she too required assistance. This was best illustrated in crayon play in which he demanded that the female therapist guide his hand as he drew, and he reciprocated by guiding her hand when she drew. We saw evidence that he was the target of his mother's rage, in that he cringed as if he anticipated annihilation whenever he was approached. On the other hand, his guiltless aggressivity was evidenced by his smiling, laughing attack on others. Thus he presented the picture of a helpless (but omnipotent) child whose every need must be fulfilled without his asking; a child to whom any physical approach may mean annihilation; a child who acted on unhostile aggressive impulses without restraint or shame.

TINA T.

Tina T. (born 1-19-57, age 3 years, 3 months at start of therapy) was the first of three children, the product of a normal pregnancy and delivery, and weighed 5½ pounds at birth. Although the immediate post-partum period was uneventful, she was from the very beginning a "feeding problem." At an early age she was fascinated with lights and by three months had developed what her father called a "thousand-yard stare." She showed no interest in people and would spend hours gazing at her hands, "wiggling her fingers like worms." At seven months of age she sat alone, and by ten months she was standing without support. From the seventh month onward she developed the habit of supporting herself on hands and knees while bumping her buttocks against the mattress, apparently oblivious of her surroundings. She did this most of the day and for periods at night. Although no particular reaction to sound or music was reported, she had unusual sensitivity in many other sensory areas. She liked to look at lamps but shaded her eyes from the light outdoors, even on a gray day. She disliked sand and grass but liked to walk on smooth floors and the asphalt driveway. At 15 months she began crawling about the house, licking the walls in certain favored

areas, licking a book, and thumping her head against a bookcase. She mouthed everything she came in contact with, being
especially fond of cords and wires. At 15 months she said
"dada" and "mama." Forcible weaning was attempted at 18
months; this failed and resulted in total and prolonged rejection of all forms of solid food. However, she plucked and ate
leaves from a bush and would chew on anything as long as it
was not food. At 21 months she began walking, and at 25
months toilet training was attempted, without success. In our
initial contact with her, her peculiar way of relating to people
was striking. At times she was quite uninterested. At times
she liked to play at running away and being caught by her
parents. She resented any attention visitors paid to her sister
but disliked being picked up herself. She was terribly frightened by groups of people, as in grocery stores. Except when
rocking in her crib, which she preferred when at all anxious,
she seemed interested in people in a cautious way but was very
hesitant about actually mixing in with them in any social
sense; she was seldom truly oblivious. The person to whom
she related most warmly was a colored maid who came once a
week.

Tina's Mother

Tina's mother (Georgia Harper) was an only child, whose
father was imprisoned for larceny (he drove a get-away car)
when Georgia was two years old. Her mother divorced him at
the insistence of the maternal grandmother. Georgia, her
mother, and a maternal aunt lived with the grandmother for
the next twelve years. When Georgia was nine years old, her
father was released from prison to enter the armed services,
and although there were several meetings between him and
Georgia, no feeling of closeness developed. In her early childhood, "bad behavior" was taken as a sure sign of "becoming
like father" and was strongly condemned. When Georgia was

sent to the store, the family carefully counted the change when she returned to be sure that she was not falling into her father's ways. Grandmother ruled the home and induced sufficient guilt in all those near her to prevent their leaving. Georgia's mother suffered unending criticism for having married against grandmother's wishes. She willingly submitted to this verbal abuse, and when it abated, she found herself another unsatisfactory mate (an alcoholic), as if to renew the cycle.

Shame and guilt accompanied Georgia in all her peer relationships. The family expected her to devote herself to her grandmother and sent her to college to equip her better for this role. In this situation Georgia found a new sense of freedom which she utilized to the maximum, but not including sexual intercourse. Shortly after graduation she dated a boy who overrode her objections to sex, raped her, and got her pregnant. She had an abortion at grandmother's insistence. Subsequently, she met her husband, began dating and having intercourse with him. During a trip to Texas to meet his parents, Mr. T. proposed marriage. She felt he was only being chivalrous and attempted to dissuade him, even to the extent of confessing the rape, pregnancy, and subsequent abortion. This only spurred him to greater insistence, and so they were married.

Tina's Father

Tina's father, a major in the Marines, is the son of a tax assessor in a Mississippi town and has a brother seven years his senior. The family operated under a sort of feudal system, wherein "the eldest son inherits all," which led to unusual rivalry between the brothers. His mother became deaf shortly after his birth, and Mr. T. has had the rigors of his delivery related to him many times. His mother is described as prissy and bird-like in her mannerisms, and she is shocked by modern attitudes towards sex. When he asked about his own origin, she told him that he "grew in the garden." She had strong ideas about vegetables, "crammed them down his throat," and he has had a strong aversion to them ever since. His mother repeatedly told him that she had wanted a girl, and he recalls the intense inferiority feelings he suffered in his peer relationships. His older brother married a Northern girl and moved into the family home. There was constant bickering between his brother and wife, and Mr. T. took a dim view of marriage in consequence. He attended a college in another state and was in the ROTC. An uncle who was a Marine officer, and whom he admired, influenced him to go into the Marine Corps.

Mr. T. entered marriage with some misgivings but felt it was "the proper thing to do." He is aware of his wife's profound dependency needs and feels that it is somehow up to him to fulfill them. Because of this sense of guilty responsibility, he is neither able to leave her nor to express his anger at her for the frustration of his own unrecognized dependency needs. In order to cope with this chronic frustration and anger without overt expression, he "chivalrously" withdraws into his books, models, and other hobbies, and communication between the two is very limited. He is adequately assertive in the company of males, in the structured routine of the Marine Corps, but in social situations tends to withdraw to himself. He excuses himself on the grounds that he is not too well liked by people, which may be related to the fact that he is given to "sounding off" in an angry and aggressive way.

The Family

Mr. T. failed to make honeymoon plans and expressed a desire to "sign in" at his new post immediately after marriage. Mrs. T. complied and they set up housekeeping in a "dirty old trailer" while awaiting post housing. Soon there ensued a three-week period of non-communication, during which his squadron was grounded, and he spent the entire time eating, sleeping, and reading. Mrs. T. dealt with this by attempting to do the same thing—making his interests her own. This went from reading novels, to designing and flying model airplanes, to stock market speculation, to coin and stamp collecting, to reading stories of World War I aviation; although there was little or no communication between them, they *were* both doing the same thing. When Tina was conceived, Mr. T. became chronically angry and spent his free time for the next two months at a friend's home. The pregnancy was accompanied by frequent nausea and vomiting, but delivery was uneventful. While she was in the hospital, Mr. T. visited once a day, seemed ill at ease, and showed no overt interest in the infant; when they returned from the hospital, he seemed totally uninterested.

Tina was a most difficult infant; she slept poorly, cried a great deal, and was a severe feeding problem. When she was three weeks old, father left for helicopter school for three months. He was unhappy about this, for he preferred flying jets. (It was ultimately learned that he had landed "wheels up" on one occasion and experienced several other close calls; this may indicate some unconscious suicidal impulses resulting from the home conflict.) Once helicopter school was complete the family took a vacation trip to Texas in spite of Tina's difficulties. Her crying, sleeplessness, and eating difficulties increased and they had to seek medical help along the way. Mrs. T. felt an implied criticism from each doctor to the effect that she was not feeding her child adequately (Mrs. T.'s mother had constantly given her vitamins so that she would not be thin like her father's family). Mrs. T. made constant heroic efforts to feed the child; one doctor suggested 18 bottles a day, and this was dutifully attempted. In Texas, Tina developed the persistent blank look which father described as a "thousand-yard stare."

After their return to North Carolina, Mr. T. soon became

ill with pneumonia and was hospitalized for five weeks. After his recovery, he made up his lost flying time, but within a month was returned to the hospital for treatment of infectious mononucleosis. During this time Mrs. T. was left with the full burden of moving to a new house and of caring for Tina, who was now bumping and rocking most of the night and was still a severe feeding problem. Shortly after Mr. T. was discharged from the hospital, his wife became pregnant again, and he reacted by avoiding her. For three weeks he stayed at the Officers' Club drinking after work instead of going home; he called this "giving her the Happy Hour treatment." Then he again began building model airplanes, which occupied all his free time. When Tina was 20 months old, still a sleeping and eating problem, uncommunicative and untrained for bladder and bowels, Eva was born. Following her birth, father became an avid stamp and coin collector.

At 26 months of age, Tina was admitted to the base hospital for study for two weeks. Her already disturbed behavior became even more regressed, and Mr. T. became more aware of his responsibilities as a father. He devoted a good deal of time to the child for a while, but was soon sent on a "good will tour" by the Corps and was away for a month. Considerable dissatisfaction with the marriage became evident, and separation was discussed. Mr. T. toyed with the idea of divorce, but felt that it was his duty to remain "for the sake of the children"; he also gave his wife's immaturity as a reason for preserving the marriage.

A temporary solution was offered by an approaching eighteen-month tour of duty overseas; dependents had to remain at home. Mr. T. hoped that during this period his wife would mature and become a more adequate mother. Prior to his departure, Tina was definitively evaluated at North Carolina Memorial Hospital, therapy for Tina and Mrs. T. arranged, and a third child conceived. At this point, Tina was refusing all foods except liquids from a bottle. She was sitting on her heels and rocking the entire night, licking the wall and bumping her head against a favorite bookcase. She was not talking, and was not bladder or bowel trained.

Course of Therapy with Tina

Originally, Tina was brought in by her mother and dumped on the floor, where she remained unless forcibly jarred out of her withdrawn state. She reached for and found any non-edible object and mouthed it continually. She soiled and wet herself without concern. She ate none of the food offered. She behaved as if oblivious of the other children and did not cry when she was bumped hard enough to hurt. If an adult paid attention to her, she got up, ran to a wire, light socket, wall hinge, or any fixed but protruding object, and mouthed it while looking at the adult teasingly. When one tried to remove her from the object, she behaved as if this were a game and clung to the object in a playful but determined manner.

After a time she began watching the other children and soon was imitating their actions and affect. If a child ran from wall to wall laughing, she would rise from the floor and replicate the action, gestures and sound; her affect, however, was empty and purely imitative. After 6–8 weeks she began her teasing game on entering the playroom, searching for something in-appropriate to put in her mouth, and drawing the attention of adults to her; she obviously enjoyed the struggle to remove the object from her mouth. She now became interested in putting her hand into the boys' pants and fondling the penis. At first the boys allowed her to play with the penis as she wished, but later they objected and struggled with her. She seemed to enjoy this struggle, too, and her intense drive to maintain this contact resulted in much scuffling. She seemed perplexed when the boys responded to her behavior by attack-ing her.

Her imitative activity increased, and soon she was seeking out other children to mimic. She enjoyed ring-around-a-rosy and chase games. When Annaletta was rough towards her she laughed with pleasure. At first she paid little attention to her mother's presence or absence, but later cried soon after mother left or if she were late in returning to pick her up; she also cried when other children left the room to go to the toilet. Later she began crying when other children struck at her, and after some six months of therapy, "bawled" when she was hit. When Annaletta was absent from the group, Tina's mood was quite subdued.

Feeding / Tina refused to be fed from a cup, and so a nursing bottle was provided. She was ecstatic over this and lay in the therapist's arms like an infant, clenching her fists and waving her arms and legs around like a little baby. She delighted in toying with the bottle and pushing it away. It became evident that her purpose was to avoid being fed. We suspected that in this play she was reliving her experience of being force-fed and was attempting to master it. We therefore made no attempt to force the nipple into her mouth, but rather permitted this playfully negativistic activity. At least twenty minutes of every session was spent in this way. She would climb into an adult's lap, assume the infantile position, and make noises like a small, happy baby. She periodically stopped the play, turned over on her abdomen, and kicked like a little baby, or climbed over one's shoulder as if to be burped. Gradually this kind of play diminished and she began drinking milk from the bottle —just a few swallows at first, and finally all the milk. Soothing, playful, loving sounds were made by the adult therapist while "feeding the baby" in this manner. If this play were interrupted too soon, she cried and clung to the worker until diverted into other activities. Eventually she requested both cup and bottle and began experimenting with drinking from the cup. When she had emptied the cup, she would refill it from the bottle; however, she always wanted to have the bottle available. Praise and joy were expressed over her attempts to drink from the cup and no criticism offered when she spilled. We also noted that she put small bits of cookie into her mouth and later ate pieces of candy.

Bowel and Bladder / Mother's method of diapering Tina included two diapers, a pair of regular pants and a pair of waterproof panties. These were so tightly applied that it seemed impossible for the child to know when she had soiled herself. We suggested that mother use a single loose-fitting diaper, and permit Tina to soil at will. Tina showed obvious pleasure in "discovering" her excretory functions. She announced "wet," stood up, and in a happy, exhibitionistic manner, wet her pants. She wanted them changed immediately and would not permit herself to be taken from the room while being changed. She later changed herself, and finally requested "potty" for both urination and defecation.

Language / Initially Tina said nothing and her "noises" were non-communicative. Later her gestures and noises were obvious mimicry and attempts to communicate. She ultimately began considerable babbling and then saying a few words. Her gestures seemed to be an imitation of mother's flirtatious manner.

Aggression / When first brought into the group, Tina responded with bewilderment when she was the object of aggression. Later she cried when hurt but made no effort to get out of the way when attacked. At times a sort of masochism was noted: She would lie on the floor "invitingly," so that the other children attacked her. She then raised her head in a pleading and tearful way toward the adult, as though to invite cuddling and protection. Subsequently she began withdrawing from attacks made by other children and later began to protest and make "pushing away" gestures when attacked. In running games in which she was being chased, either playfully or hostilely, she ran behind the adult and used the adult to fend off the attack. She finally defended herself vigorously when attacked by pushing the assailant away, crying, and seeking adult protection. Her own aggression was manifested by brief tantrums followed by seductive behavior towards the nearest adult.

Masturbation / During the first eight months of therapy

Tina was compulsively interested in the boys' genitals, much more so than in her own, but eventually she did indulge in masturbation for long periods. She usually hid while doing this, as if ashamed, but when the other children observed her, they attempted to inspect and touch her genitals, too. This upset her, especially when they became rough.

To recapitulate, Tina's behavior during early therapy consisted of isolated mouthing of objects, determined non-feeding, playing with male genitals, and ultimately masturbation. Each of these acts had a provocative, teasing quality, as if both to discharge anxiety and to gain the attention of the female therapists. We may speculate that such behavior had reliably evoked some response from her mother.

Interaction of Tina T. Family

Mrs. T. is an immature, guilt-laden mother who felt a debt of gratitude to the man who had married her in spite of (perhaps because of) her "badness," a mother whose pattern of behavior included parading her guilts in order to obtain punishment and forgiveness, and thus maintain a dependency relationship with people who might potentially mother her. For Mrs. T., Tina is the "bad self" who needs punishment but also needs complete dependence upon the mother. In her relationship with Tina, Mrs. T. takes for herself the role of the omnipotent, forgiving mother, but through identification with Tina she becomes at the same time a repentant, forgiven child, thus reconstituting all elements of the former symbiotic relationship with her own mother.

Major T.'s dependency wishes are similarly conflictual and are dealt with by identification with the "bad" female whom he rescues, then abandons. His hostility towards females (either as mother or girl child) is kept out of awareness by isolation and compulsive hobbies. He is a man whose sexual identity is adequate in the structured routine of the Marine Corps, but this identity becomes confused in the family and social situation. It is likely that Tina represents the female child his mother wanted, whom he rescues and then abandons.

Tina's behavior in the group was that of a child with primary autism who made contact with mothering figures by mouthing of inedible objects in a provocative, teasing way. Relatedness developed when the mothering person attempted to remove the object from Tina's mouth. It seems that the feeding struggle was a traumatic experience for the child and thus a fixating experience. We understood the early feeding situation in terms of the mother's fear that if Tina got really hungry, she might become upset and not eat. Therefore Tina was always fed before she was hungry, so that feeding was not associated with satisfaction of a hunger need, but rather in terms of aggression. We concluded that the tenacious play of mouthing inedible objects, genital play with others and with herself, were patterned responses aimed at mastering the early unpleasurable experience of being fed. Accordingly, we attempted to produce a corrective emotional experience [7] in the feeding situation. We gave Tina permission *not* to eat and instead indulged her need to ward off the dangerous bottle. This resulted in her emergence from the autistic phase of development and entry into a rather happy symbiotic phase, and ultimately into steps towards separation-individuation. As these developmental steps proceeded, the interaction between child and parents, however, continued to be one in which Tina was the "bad child" who needed protection, punishment, and dependency upon the mother, and the "injured female" who needs rescuing by the male (father) and is subsequently abandoned. The bulk of therapy with Tina consisted of dealing with her constant attempts to provoke similar reactions from the female and male therapists.

7. F. Alexander (1954), Some quantitative aspects of psychoanalytic technique, *Journal of the American Psychoanalytic Association*, 2:685–701.

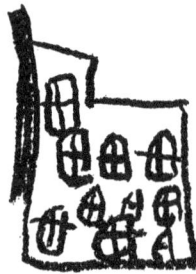

BOB B.

Bob B. (born 7-4-55, age 4 years, 10 months at start of therapy) was a full-term child, delivered by cesarean section because of placenta previa. He breathed spontaneously at birth and weighed 8 pounds, 1 ounce. Mother cannot recall specific dates regarding his early development and answers questions by saying, "He was normal like other children." At about four years of age, mother realized that Bob was behaving oddly, and went to the neighbors to find out if they had noted any changes. They informed her of their observations of his peculiar actions, and over the next six months, mother became increasingly aware of this bizarre behavior. In our initial contact with mother her complaints were that Bob paid no attention to her, would not obey her, and did not even seem to hear her; he would spend hours twirling objects, raptly listening to television commercials, and switching lights on and off. He did not sleep well and would awaken her in the early morning by switching her bed lamp on and off. He had a singsong voice and most of what he said made no sense. She found this behavior embarrassing, and because of it she withdrew from most of her social activities.

Bob's Mother

Bob's Mother (Jean Smith) was the third of four children (two boys and two girls) whose machinist father loved to putter around the farm, and whose mother was very active in church and community affairs. Jean was born and reared in a small town adjoining a larger one and had a strong feeling of being from "the wrong side of the tracks." Her parents had widely divergent social ambitions but never quarreled about this openly. Jean also emphasizes that she lived her early childhood during the Depression, when money was tight. Her sister, eight years older, was the family pet, and Jean resented having to wear her hand-me-down clothes. A brother, two years younger, suffered from asthma and Jean recalls her envy of the attention he got during his attacks. Her earliest memory is of a neighbor's house burning, and she recalls nightmares filled with the crackling noise of fire; her terror brought mother to the bed to comfort her. Jean vividly describes the wretchedness of the children from her town who attended the neighboring city school and relates with great affect her intense feelings of inferiority and her envy of those fortunate enough to have been born in the select city. She gleefully describes how a girl from "the wrong side of the tracks" was once elected to office in the high school and marks it as a great victory over the "snobs." After high school she attended a strict church school for a year and the state university for two years. The freedom at the University was exciting, but for unexplained reasons she quit after her third year and went to work. She dated her boss, 12 years her senior, and after two years of dating they were married. This marriage was the culmination of her life's ambitions: her husband was financially and socially successful in the envied town adjoining her home. It was for her the fulfilment of the Cinderella fantasy in all details.

Bob's Father

Bob's father (Bob Sr.) is the fourth in a family of five children. His father, who died when he was 14 years old, had hypertension and "drank heavily, but was not alcoholic." His mother, an asthmatic, is still living. A brother, four years younger, was killed in World War II at the age of 23. Mr. B. recalls that his brothers and sisters all preferred outdoor work, while he preferred to putter about the house helping his mother, even though he was ridiculed for this. He also recalls being ill frequently and feels he enjoyed invalidism. At age 13, he underwent a T & A (which was repeated after his marriage) and had an undescended testicle removed at the same time. On three occasions he had serious doubts about his ability to learn: twice he dropped back to a lower grade briefly, then resumed his normal class position; on the third occasion he withdrew from college for a week, dropped chemistry, and then returned to his studies. It is noteworthy that he graduated with honors from high school and was second in his class at college. Following graduation he took a job with a local company which he has held ever since, but with relatively little advancement. He dated a girl regularly for four years, but she dropped him when he refused, on moral grounds, to gratify her sexual wishes. He then began dating his present wife. He has been constantly plagued by problems relating to sex and has profound guilt feelings over fantasies about women other than his wife. His first episode of clinical depression occurred following a New Year's Eve party in which he drank more than usual and indulged in unplanned (and unsatisfactory) intercourse with his wife. Since then, he has approached sex in a highly compulsive and ritualistic way; at least 18 hours of planning are necessary in preparation. In addition, he feels intense guilt over his feelings about his wife's social and intellectual status, which he considers beneath his own. He becomes irritated about the fact that his children deprive him of his wife's attention, and this, too, produces feelings of guilt.

Mr. B. suffered from a great many physical ailments following marriage, primarily sore throats, colds, and back trouble. He ultimately had some tonsillar tags removed, with some improvement. According to his wife, the medical expenses during their marriage amounted to $700 to $1,000 yearly. At first the marriage evoked some complications in social and emotional adjustment, since his friends were considerably older than hers. After 1½ years of marriage, Mrs. B. gave birth to a baby girl. Pregnancy and delivery were without complications, and the child's development and adjustment seem quite normal.

Mr. B. had always dreamed of a permanent home, and so they built one in 1953, when they had been married five years. Two years later, at his wife's insistence, she conceived again. The pregnancy was uncomplicated until the seventh month, when painless bleeding occurred. This did not recur until term, at which time a cesarean section was performed because of placenta previa. Bob Jr. was a healthy baby, who was carefully examined by the doctors and pronounced normal. It took his mother a long time to recover from the surgery, and she describes a moderately severe post-partum depression which lasted three months. The depression ended when she released the maid, weaned Bob from the breast, and assumed her household duties. Mr. B. began experiencing moods of depression shortly after Bob's birth, and when the child was six months old, suffered a severe depressive reaction, for which he was hospitalized for several months and received electroconvulsive therapy. He suffered a second break about a year later, and a third one when Bob was nearly four. During these 3½ years, Mrs. B. had to assume all the responsibilities for the home and children, while at the same time, Mr. B. required almost constant mothering. She describes long hours of listening to his physical complaints and reassuring him of his goodness and of his being needed. It seems clear that she was totally absorbed in taking care of her husband, for she is quite unable to recall any details of Bob's development during this period. During the last depressive episode, she recalls that Bob sang all the time, and states, "If he had not sung, he would not have survived his father's illness." Toward the end of this last episode, Bob's behavior became so peculiar that his mother could no longer ignore it.

Relations with her mother-in-law were also quite strained, because she felt that she was blamed for her husband's illness. She was full of unconscious rage over her bad luck. She maintained that if it were not for psychiatrists, she and her family would be well and happy. She insisted that all she wanted was a private life without psychiatrists prying into it. She denied any and all anger, and insisted that she had none, inasmuch as she was brought up to love without hate or anger. She expressed her great disappointment over Bob's difficulty, since she felt that her husband was now getting better, and if it were not for Bob's illness, they would have the life she so much desired. Mr. B. developed rigid obsessive-compulsive attitudes to deal with his conflicts and assiduously avoided expressing anger toward his family, instead spending hours "discussing" with his wife detailed plans for dealing with all current situations, however minor. Social drinking, vacation, money matters, business difficulties due to personality conflicts, handling of Bob, and "what the psychiatrist said" were obsessively dealt with at lunch time and after office hours. Bob constantly interfered with these discussions, and the need to exclude him was a source of frustration for both parents. At one time they handled this by locking him in his bedroom.

Bob

Formal psychological testing was impossible because of his inability to co-operate, but he gave the impression of having normal intelligence. The psychiatrists observed the following points: Bob had a singsong voice, and his verbalizations were irrelevant. He completely ignored people other than his mother. He was fascinated by lights and switches. Mother kept trying to persuade Bob to talk: "Say hello to the doctor. Tell him what you did this morning. Sing him that song you learned and liked. Talk to the doctor. Say goodbye to the doctor." To all this Bob gave no relevant responses. A diagnosis of psychosis was rendered by the child psychiatry staff, and treatment in the proposed group project was recommended.

Course in Therapy with Bob

Aggression / Originally Bob seemed to be extremely anxious every moment he was with us, and he handled this by intensely aggressive behavior. He seemed to be anticipating retaliation, and this may have accounted for his apparent slyness and sneakiness, which we found so provocative. At times he openly "asked" for spankings. When another child attacked him, he screamed as though he felt he was being annihilated. He aggressively attacked all objects, which he destroyed indiscriminately, and all persons except the male therapists. Tina was a special target for aggression. He was a bit wary of Mike and Walter but would hit them if their backs were turned. When Annaletta entered the group he attacked her viciously, but her retaliatory blows soon put a stop to this. We early recognized his need and wish for control, and began holding him whenever he showed signs of agitation. At first, he was held gently, but the closeness seemed to make him feel more terrified. Then he was held firmly and decisively, with arms and legs twined around him from behind. We interpreted his fear over loss of control and explained that we were supplying outer control so that he could learn to control himself and not be so scared. Initially he fought this viciously, but gradually he became aware that we were not trying to hurt him but rather help him. After several months of this he would say " 'trol Bob," asking us to control him. When he felt calmed down he would say "Bob 'trol Bob now," and we would let him go, saying that if he found he could not control himself, he should return, and we would help him again.

At this point, Bob became obsessed with a "ghost," and it seemed that gaining control of his actions permitted this fantasy to be verbalized. This was a difficult period for the parents, because Bob had great difficulty sleeping, particularly sleeping alone. We had previously discouraged his mother from sleeping with him, and his father tried to help him with his fear by lying down with him until the agitation ceased. Eventually we were able to convince father that all he needed to do was enter the room, let Bob know he was there, and perhaps sit with him a few moments. This was a terrifying time for Bob, and he was given a tranquilizer for about four months (meprobamate syrup, 800 mgm. daily). He was finally able to tell us that the ghost was himself, mother, dad, and Dr. Speers, and soon thereafter he was able to maintain good self-control in the group situation and improved self-control at home. The nightmares became less frequent and he slept uninterruptedly almost every night.

Speech / Initially Bob's speech was almost unintelligible. He misused pronouns ("you" instead of "I") and there seemed to be neologisms in his singsong speech. We were surprised to discover that he had some capacity for reality testing, when he told us that the clay was "play-like cookies," for previously he had seemed out of contact most of the time. He gave the impression of a child who, because of intense fear of his aggressive urges and the fantasied retaliation for them, had regressed to an infantile state in order to discharge the aggression safely. As his behavior became controllable, his speech became clearer; he began using sentences of five to six words, which were understandable and communicative.

Feeding / Bob's initial attitude toward food in the group was highly aggressive. He devoured everything he could get his hands on and destroyed what he could not eat. When he was encouraged to try the nursing bottle, he climbed onto an adult lap and allowed himself to be fed like a baby. He subsequently became very well-behaved about eating, and was able to wait while the food was being prepared; he also gave food to the adults and other children in the group. Initially there was a problem of his biting other children in the group and chewing inedible objects. Both subsided as his anxiety decreased, and ultimately a type of ruminative chewing occurred only while he was daydreaming.

Sexual behavior / Bob was delighted with Tina's interest in his genitals, and stood quite still when she reached into his pants to touch his penis. He often took his penis out, looked at it and put it back in his trousers. When Annaletta entered the group, his destructive behavior was still at its height (or only declining slowly) and was augmented during her early participation. When Annaletta took off her clothing and danced around in the nude, Bob did likewise. He tore off his clothes and did whatever Annaletta did. He urinated on the floor, exhibited his penis, and generally showed off to the females in the room. The other boys became upset over his behavior, and began grabbing and pulling at his penis, which seemed to discourage this exhibitionistic behavior. However, during the first year and one-half of therapy, Bob still urinated on the floor when he was severely frustrated.

Interaction of Bob B. Family

Bob Sr. is a bright and potentially capable "mamma's boy," whose marriage to Jean reconstituted his previous dependency relationship with his mother. The first child (a girl) threatened this dependency, and he reacted with frequent illness, and even had a re-operation for tonsillar tags. With the birth of the second child (Bob) the rage elicited by further dependency frustration culminated in a severe depressive reaction six months later. He misidentified Bob with his own younger brother, and we speculate that Jean's pregnancy and postpartum depression may have reactivated potent childhood memories of his own mother when she was bearing the now dead brother. Mr. B.'s attempts to avert and deal with his hostility by clinging dependently to his wife, and by obsessive-compulsive behavior resulted in a barely marginal adjustment. He tried to monopolize all of her time and to exclude Bob from contact with her; this produced intense guilt which he dealt with by periodic oversolicitousness toward his son.

Jean described her marriage as extremely successful during the first year or so, the culmination of her hopes and dreams. Her husband's reaction following the birth of the first child threatened the defensive structure which she had built to avoid feelings of inadequacy or inferiority. We speculate that her insistence upon a second child was a misguided effort to recapture the early years of her marriage. But the birth of a *male* child reactivated the hostile feelings she had experienced toward her younger brother because of the loss of dependency gratification from her mother. She reacted to the resulting ambivalence by forming a symbiotic union with Bob. In addition, there is little doubt that Mrs. B. perceived Bob's birth as a prime factor in her husband's subsequent depression, and she had feelings of monumental rage toward this child who had wrecked her entire defensive structure. Her dependent and narcissistic needs were now frustrated, and her envy and hate of those more fortunate than herself were reactivated to a profound degree. In order to avoid becoming depressed, she used the child to express her own rage, envy, and jealousy. She clung to him tenaciously, identifying with his dependency wishes, thus vicariously gaining gratification of her own; in addition, she used him to act out her own hostile and envious feelings toward others. Thus, when Mr. B. was not at home, Mrs. B. and Bob were inseparable. Visits to stores and neighbors' homes were orgies of destructive behavior on Bob's part, and of futile efforts by his mother to control it. When his father was at home, Bob was locked in his room to prevent his interfering with the parents' frantic efforts to deal with their mutual hostility and satisfy their mutual dependency wishes. Each sought to inflict revenge and blame on the other by using Bob, who seemed always underfoot in the bathroom and parental bedroom and was a constant interruption at the table.

We speculate that in spite of the hostile interaction between father and son, the father represented to Bob a non-symbiotic object which permitted the possibility of escape from the all-engulfing relationship with mother. The father's illness and hospitalization forestalled this possibility and resulted in Bob's being totally engulfed psychologically by his mother. Bob was able to tolerate two such separations from father, but the third resulted in a rupture of his weakened ego, and a regressive psychosis ensued. It appeared as though he alternated between a sort of happy symbiosis wherein he acted out his mother's hostile wishes (gaining dependency gratification from her in return) and a type of autistic attitude, which served to maintain some separateness from mother and prevented a total loss of self. Admission into the children's group broke the symbiotic tie with mother and at the same time frustrated his attempts to withdraw autistically. The resultant anxiety was of panic proportions. Bob's sly, provocative aggressivity toward other children seemed the re-enactment of his pattern of acting out his mother's envy and rage towards others, but also was an attempt to destroy the children who interfered with symbiotic possibilities with the female therapists. His behavior toward the male therapists was cautious and provocative. He seemed to be anticipating annihilation from them, especially when he was in close contact with the female therapists. The application of consistent external controls ultimately enabled him to refrain from his destructive behavior and to verbalize his intense fears of the "ghost" and its retaliatory threats. Contact with the female therapists went through several phases: first, close physical contact which obviously stimulated him sexually; then attempts to keep the therapist fascinated by obsessive questioning (reminiscent of his parents' obsessive discussions); later he could be satisfied by minimal skin contact now and then; and ultimately he could tolerate long periods of separation from the female. With the male therapists he progressed from obvious fear of annihilation to warmth and appreciation of the controls placed upon him, then to some identification with the male role.

During the course of therapy, Bob recapitulated some of the processes of psychosexual development. First there was autistic behavior, with passive acceptance of erotic stimulation as he was held, comforted, and soothed. Concomitantly, there was voracious eating, then passive acceptance of the bottle, and the experience of being held and accepted in this manner. Then there was smearing finger-paint, crayoning, playing with clay and eating it, and wetting himself with the bubble water. Finally there was exhibitionistic behavior, nudism, "accidental" fondling of the female therapists, and voyeuristic peeping at Tina and Annaletta.

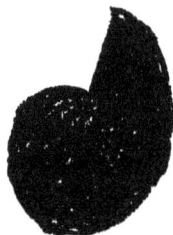

MIKE M.

Mike M. (born 4-8-56, 4 years, 1 month at start of therapy) is the oldest of three children (John, 18 months younger, and Jeannette, 3 years younger) born following an uncomplicated pregnancy and delivery. At age three, Mike's mother read a pamphlet on "autism"; she suspected that he was autistic and sought diagnostic confirmation at a large medical center six months later. She complained that Mike had always been a feeding problem and that he seemed totally oblivious of people; she was unable to make him mind or even listen to her. He was not bowel or bladder trained. His speech was bizarre and made no sense to mother. He would sit and watch television commercials or a turning phonograph record for hours. Mother's only contact with him was when she pointed out geometrical designs in a magazine or book and he repeated the name of each design for her. She stated that he was fascinated by lights and that he responded pleasantly to certain musical sounds but violently to others. She felt a complete inability to understand him, help him, or deal with him.

Mike's Mother

Mike's mother (Gloria), age 27, is the elder of two daughters born of European parents. Gloria's mother is described as "a warm, happy-go-lucky optimist who is far too trusting of others and is thus readily hurt by their ordinary behavior; a woman who needs many overt expressions of love and affection." Gloria's father is from a family of eleven children. He entered dentistry, disliked it, quit, and came to the United States from Germany during the Depression. Gloria describes him as a "perfectionist who feels that expressions of love towards a woman are unmanly." She thinks her parents' marriage was basically stable, but marred by lack of emotional communication: "Each cried out for understanding by the other, but never bothered to explain his own feelings."

When Gloria was three years old, a sister was born and intense rivalry developed. She criticizes her sister for her "immature behavior and total lack of consideration," and harshly condemns any sort of "childishness" in her sister and others.

At an early age, Gloria visited Europe with her mother and attended kindergarten in Holland where she learned to speak Dutch and German as well as English. When she returned to the United States to enter the first grade at a Catholic school, she felt shy and timid, with a sense of inferiority which she ascribed to being the daughter of a German father during the World War II years. She was also highly sensitive that her father was the custodian at the schoolhouse, and she speaks of his not having an office like the fathers of the other children. When she passed her father in the hall at school, she refused to speak to him. In college Gloria emerged somewhat from her isolation, began dating, and made some close friendships. She majored in psychology, and after graduation worked in an EEG laboratory, during which time she met her husband, a medical student at a nearby college. They began dating regularly and were married two years later.

Mike's Father

Mike's father (Edgar) was an only child. His mother is "a doormat who wallows in self-pity, and blames all her misfortunes on acts of the Lord;" his father "drinks to calm his nerves, and demands constant affection to the point of effusiveness." A paternal aunt suffered a psychotic depression and committed suicide. The paternal grandparents' attitude toward Mike's illness is "to hide him so people won't know about it, which would disgrace the entire family."

Mr. M. was not merely an only child but was the only male child on either side of the family, and thus received all the rewards and opportunities of such a situation. Upon graduation from college, he entered medical school, but failed his second year, decided he was "not suited for medicine," and quit even though he would have been permitted to repeat the year. He now works as a junior executive in a textile mill.

The Family

Mr. and Mrs. M. were married secretly after his failure in medical school, and they did not inform his parents of the marriage until after the honeymoon. This led to strained relations between Mrs. M. and her in-laws, but she combatted it by ignoring their hostile attitudes. She conceived shortly after marriage but aborted at 4½ months. Vaginal hemorrhage occurred during the third month of gestation but expulsion of the fetus did not occur until six weeks later. She was told that the fetus was normal, but the placenta abnormal. She suffered a severe reaction to this loss and five months later, when pregnant with Mike, embarked upon a stringent prenatal program of vitamins, calcium, rest, etc., to insure against a recurrence of the disaster of the first pregnancy. At term, the membranes ruptured, and when uterine contractions failed to follow, oxytocic drugs were administered. Even when she was taken to the delivery room, the contractions were not strong and were still five minutes apart. Delivery was by means of "low forceps, without difficulty." Mike breathed spontaneously, and weighed 5 pounds, 14 ounces. There were no immediate post-partum difficulties.

Mike

In the initial history, mother described Mike as a "colicky baby." In group therapy she described her barely controlled rage over feeding difficulties. Mike cried, screamed, and hollered for nearly eighteen months, and nothing she could do would alleviate the situation. When finally this behavior ceased, Mike became a passive, totally unreachable child who lay in his crib for hours without making a sound. She ultimately recalled that he gained weight at a phenomenal rate and admits that she possibly overfed him. He was quite rigid during feeding, rolling his eyes and clenching his jaws. At age five months he fell from the bathinette, but cried immediately, and had no discernible after-effects.

Mike sat up at seven months and stood up a week later. He cut his first tooth at ten months and "they sprouted like mushrooms from then on." He walked at eleven months. His mother describes a time when he would look at people and smile at them, but this soon ceased. He withdrew when other people were around. In the toddler stage, Mike would not lift his own glass until mother refused to do it for him. He then lifted the glass, but seemed frightened of it. Bowel training was a total failure when attempted at two years of age. They tried spanking and long sessions on the toilet, but to no avail. She described his leaving small deposits all over the house for her to clean up and insisted he did this to spite her. At three years of age he underwent herniorrhaphy, which frightened him, but mother insists that this produced no change other than a slight increase in tantrum behavior.

Mike's speech seemed bizarre to the parents. He repeated words correctly, but never in context. He memorized TV commercials and when asked a question, would respond with a jingle. He became preoccupied with all sorts of tubes, phonograph records, certain songs, and twirling objects. He would play for hours by himself without uttering a sound or noting others and during this time would twirl an object or himself. He was fascinated with geometric designs and the only contact mother could get with him was to sit down and teach him the names of such figures as triangle, star, diamond, trapezoid, and the like; he would correctly name each figure after such a session. He completely ignored strangers and other children but would sit and watch his younger brother, John. Although fascinated with the commercials on TV, he had no interest in the program. He enjoyed turning lights on and off. He would not mind his mother and seemed oblivious of danger. Despite these many unusual characteristics, Mike's parents did not seek help for him until 3½ years of age, partly because a local doctor had said he was a genius, and partly because the paternal grandparents said he was not different from what his father had been like as a young child.

Mike was evaluated psychiatrically in February, 1960, and was given a diagnosis of "infantile autism, but with a better prognosis than usual." His intelligence was estimated to be average to superior. During the re-evaluation at North Carolina Memorial Hospital, observers were impressed with his autistic behavior and the bizarreness of his language, which was unrelated to reality except when he was naming geometric designs. It was noted, however, that he exhibited some interest in people if the person slowly intruded on him without interfering with his activities. He had also a certain exhibitionistic attitude which was hard to define but which enhanced the prognosis in the opinion of several psychiatrists. The diagnosis offered was "childhood psychosis with autistic behavior (probably not primary autism)." Treatment in the proposed psychotic children's group was recommended.

Course in Therapy with Mike

Aggression / Mike's initial contact with the group was very cautious. He did not look at the other children or at the adults, but occupied himself with objects, which he would twirl continuously. He was fascinated by the phonograph and would watch the record spin for long periods of time. He routinely defecated in his pants on entering the room and at times would lie on his back, roll over the feces in his pants, and with a dreamy look on his face seem to be indulging in revery. Periodically, he would utter incongruous words such as "beachballs," "tubes," and "Papa bear"; he kept out of the group activities and remained oblivious of the other children for weeks. He ate what food was offered to him but was always by himself while actually eating. When we took movies of the children he became fearful and excited and threw toys at the flood-lamps.

One of the first behavioral changes noted was his interest in the mirror; he would go and stand by it for long periods, examining his mouth and teeth. When he found his uvula, he seemed ecstatic; he went around looking in the adults' mouths, and then announced, "two penises." But as the other children gradually became more aggressive, he became more frightened. When attacked, he would run to a male therapist and in obvious panic "melt" into him. He attempted to avoid the other children, but when this failed he went into violent tantrums, falling on the floor, and kicking and biting himself. We held him during these times and attempted to reassure him that we would protect him. When protection failed, he lashed out bitterly at the adults. Ultimately he seemed to sense the need to counterattack; after waiting for an opportunity, he would violently attack any child who had previously attacked him. This necessitated a good deal of intervention and comforting. Thus Mike's aggression went through several phases; bland passivity and unawareness of being attacked; panicky flights from aggression directed against him; uncontrolled rage directed only at himself; diffuse aggression directed outward, but indiscriminately; outward aggression directed at individuals, but still uncontrollable; controlled, retaliatory aggression, restricted to an actual aggressor; finally frustration aggression of a controlled type, i.e., if he did not get what he wanted right away, he exhibited angry behavior toward the frustrating person in the form of moderate slapping. This later changed to pouting or defecating when frustrated. When these behaviorisms were identified as indicating anger, Mike would direct the anger outward again, but now toward inanimate objects—the inflated clown, crackers, or a ball, etc. After two years of therapy, Mike retaliated when attacked, but in a controlled way which did not require intervention. He pouted at times but no longer defecated when frustrated.

Sexual behavior / Mike seemed intrigued when Tina fondled his genitals, and permitted this to some extent. He observed Annaletta undressed and grabbed at her genitals vigorously. In an exhibitionistic way which revealed his fascination, he informed his parents, "All the boys have a penis, and so does Tina, but Annaletta does not." He frequently had erections and lolled over the female workers, attempting to fondle their breasts. He insisted that Tina take off her panties and talked of girls with no pants. He paid much attention to the fact that "Tina has an anus," but was unwilling to admit she had no penis. Eventually we "decoded" his talk about beachballs, tubes, white pants, and babies, which referred to seeing his mother undressed at the beach when she was pregnant with Jeannette; her skin was untanned where it had been covered by the bathing suit, and he perceived this as "white pants." In this connection, his interest in inflating and particularly deflating beach balls and tubes likewise became intelligible. His obsessive self-reassurance that boys and girls are alike with respect to the anus, and his denial that the girls lacked a penis seemed to indicate intense castration anxiety. For a while, the presence of the uvula seemed to reassure him, but this faded. For nearly two years he remained enthusiastic about looking at Tina and trying to feel her anus. Whenever he saw Tina's genitals he would close his eyes, run to a male therapist, and bury his head in the therapist's lap. He exhibitionistically bragged about his knowledge of penises and seemed delighted over the size of his father's.

Toilet training / Initially, Mike soiled himself as soon as he entered the therapy room. This combined an aggressive act (a way of keeping others away from him) and an autoerotic act, in that he was observed to indulge in revery during and after it. He later used soiling primarily to express anger and frustration. However, he noted the attention the other children were getting by being taken out of the room to go to the toilet, and this subsequently became a way for him to get attention

and to get away from the other children. He used this obsessively but it did result in his becoming toilet trained. It was
obvious that he withheld feces until he got to the Clinic and
then made several prolonged trips to the bathroom in the
company of the female worker. When this was pointed out to
him he responded by pouting and soiled himself angrily, but
this soon stopped and he shortly became completely trained.

Language / From incongruous, explosive, and exhibitionistic phrases, Mike gradually progressed to the development of
communicative speech. He now makes known his wants, and
will respond to questions. He gradually revealed his fantasy
about the beach ball and its significance regarding pregnancy.
Periodically, he communicates with other children, but rather
tentatively. He now uses pronouns correctly. At first he communicated only fantasy material but at the end of two years
was talking about current reality phenomena as well. It seems
that his speech, like his learning in general, had been fixated
on past traumata (and related fantasies) which he had been
unable to resolve, and he subsequently related all things to
that trauma and fixation. The development of less stereotyped object relations, and the control of aggression, permitted
verbalization of the fantasies. As distortions and misunder-
standings were clarified, reality-oriented abilities appeared.

Interaction of Mike M. Family

Mike's parents are people who "play at" being adults. Each
admits some childishness in himself, but, believing in the
maturity of the spouse, feels safe and comfortable. They have a
strong need to deny dependency wishes, feeling that such desires are infantile and unacceptable. Except for the display of
love and affection, all human emotions are approached in a
detached, intellectual manner. Each member of the family is
supposed to present only mature behavior at all times and to
disdain all childlike desires. Anger, being a threat to love, is

disavowed. The mutual dissatisfactions in the marriage are left unexpressed, for fear of disrupting the intense mutual dependency, and so as to display a façade of complete, idyllic harmony to the outside world and to themselves. They displace their mutual frustration and conflicts onto Mike and attempt to solve them through him.

Mrs. M. had to see herself as a sophisticated, intellectual person with profound scorn for the childishness she saw in others. She wanted to be recognized as "mature" by authority figures, and with this in mind, her demeanor was smooth and well-modulated. Her anger was also rigidly controlled, but when it did break through, she quickly restored her composure, and then in a calm, intellectual manner verbally demolished her adversaries by deprecating their childishness. She identified Mike as her own infantile self: he gained what she had forced herself to give up. In addition, she misidentified him as her spoiled, infantile sister, and she constantly admonished him to "grow up." It was essential for Mrs. M. to maintain a symbiotic relationship with Mike in order to gratify vicariously her own dependency wishes; through identification, she gained the affection she so strongly desired. Verbal contact between Mike and his mother (on a pseudo-communicative level) occurred only when she saw him as her former self, an intelligent, exhibitionistic child; she taught him, and he recited, the names of colors, geometric designs, letters, and numbers.

Mike was identified by his father as the pampered self that is both longed for and disdained as being too similar to the depreciated paternal grandfather (who "drinks to calm his nerves" and demands a great show of affection). Mr. M. presented himself as a "big wheel," an omnipotent male with whom the child could not identify, such perfection being unattainable. His wife added to this by aggrandizing him and depreciating Mike.

Thus Mike was caught in a bind: his parents demanded

maturity on the one hand but encouraged infantility on the other. He was goaded toward a goal of perfection but identified as "bad," "incompetent," and "sick." He was constantly manipulated and overstimulated by his mother, but could not express his frustration, for fear of abandonment. The pathological relationship between Mike and his mother began at birth and reached a climax at eighteen months, when his brother was born. At this time Mike became autistic. The family was able to avoid perception of this serious disturbance for two years, but after the birth of the third child, Mike had even more severe regressive symptoms, which could not be denied.

Mike entered the group in a state of autistic withdrawal but occasionally showed an obvious interest in people. Once his defense was penetrated, and the anxiety dealt with, Mike presented the various roles assigned to him by his parents: the intelligent child who could name geometric designs correctly; the infantilized child who achieved the needed symbiotic union with omnipotent parents by "melting into" adults; the bad exhibitionistic child who behaved in a stupid, bizarre manner. In a fragmentary way, he alluded to specific traumatic experiences and fantasies by uttering certain key words, illustrating his anxiety about sexual differences, pregnancy, and babies.

In therapy Mike experienced relationships with females who had no need to infantilize him, to use him for their own exhibitionistic purposes, nor to depreciate him as a male child. He was exposed to males who did not have to compete with him, and who thus permitted him to identify with them. As a result, Mike was able to separate himself as an entity and to gain a concept of himself as an adequate male. He could compete with boys of his own age and size and gain pleasure from the experience of winning at times. He still, however, used his old patterns of behavior when approaching a new situation but could deal with it realistically after a reasonable period of time.

ANNALETTA A.

Annaletta A. (born 2-19-56, age 4½ years at start of therapy) is the youngest of four children of a 34-year-old, twice divorced woman who depends on the Welfare Department for support. Mrs. A. intimates that Annaletta was conceived in an extramarital affair while her second husband was in prison. The three older children were taken from Mrs. A. by the DPW on grounds of "child neglect," before Annaletta was two years old. She was permitted to remain with her mother because "no one would take Anna." The maternal grandmother, who lives in the home with Mrs. A. and Annaletta, works in a local hosiery mill, but does not contribute to the support of the other two; if she did, they would lose Welfare support. In our contact with Mrs. A., it has become clear that she has had a symbiotic relationship with her mother as well as with her daughter.

Mrs. A. makes a marginal adjustment as an ambulatory schizophrenic, and her recollection of Annaletta's early childhood is sketchy and inconstant. She refused to submit the autobiography which each mother was requested to write. However, we do have reports from other sources, which give some idea of the child's early difficulties. Annaletta was seen at three years of age by her family physician, who diagnosed grand mal seizures, and treated her with phenobarbital. The seizures stopped, but 3 months later he referred her to a local hospital because of behavioral symptoms. There they obtained the history that the child had fallen down several steps shortly before the seizures began. She appeared to be out of contact with her surroundings, paid no attention to her mother, and was unable to get along with other children. Although she had previously learned to talk and could sing several songs, she now said only "daddy" and "mommy." The anticonvulsant medication was continued, although physical examination and electroencephalogram had not indicated any neurological abnormality; a subsequent EEG has also been reported as normal. She was diagnosed as having "infantile schizophrenia, due probably to organic brain damage."

At four years of age, Annaletta was seen in the child guidance clinic of the Mental Health Center in her community, where a somewhat different history was obtained. Here it was reported that she had had seizures since birth, had never talked except for one or two words, and was sensitive to noises (she would, for instance, cover her ears when she heard water running in the bathtub). At that time, she was not toilet trained, and she played with her feces after depositing them on the floor. When she was frustrated, she would have severe tantrums. The mother also described "laughing spells" in which Annaletta would laugh, without provocation, for periods of four to five minutes. She slept poorly at night and at times would point to the wall, reacting as though something were there—this was felt to represent hallucination. The psychiatrist at the clinic noted her extreme hyperactivity, impulsivity, irritability, restlessness, and poorly organized behavior and felt that this indicated diffuse brain damage. Because she related to people, it was thought that she could not have schizophrenia or autism. They noted that she communicated not by using words, but by means of gestures, facial grimaces, and bizarre sounds. Deafness was not considered likely and it was predicted that language would eventually develop. Her intelligence was estimated to about IQ 50. The final diagnosis was "brain damage of diffuse character." Institutionalization was recommended.

Mrs. A. was dissatisfied with the recommendation of the Mental Health Clinic and requested an appointment at North Carolina Memorial Hospital when Annaletta was 4½ years old. This time she gave the history that at one year of age, Annaletta had been ill for several days with a high fever, had fallen from a chair, and had had a convulsion. The "seizures" subsequent to this event, as described by her mother, were hard to picture as being anything more than tantrums. Interviewing Mrs. A. was a perplexing process, since it was extremely difficult for her to communicate even quite simple facts. She would wander off onto other subjects, vaguely harangue against her mother, the DPW, or other doctors, and persistently demand to be told what medicine to give Anna. Her facial expression and demeanor suggested intense anger with impending loss of control.

Annaletta was found to be an equally peculiar and perplexing child. She was amazingly dextrous and manipulated both large and small objects with remarkable speed and accuracy. She was continuously active physically, her restlessness suggesting intense anxiety. She used a few words in a forceful way, but they were clipped and jerky, stereotyped and difficult to understand; she seemed to use them for expression of affect, not for communication. On the other hand, her gestures and facial expressions appeared communicative and potentially meaningful. It appeared as though she was too "driven" to try to bother with language; her needs were so urgent and intense that to try to communicate verbally would only frustrate her by further delay. It must be emphasized that she was not a withdrawn child: her wish to interact and communicate was unmistakable. It is interesting to compare her frustration in this regard to her mother's marked difficulty in verbal communication. Though mother does not lack words, she uses them in a confusing way, and gestural communication may represent a "private language" which is less ambiguous, but difficult for outsiders to "decode."

It was difficult to evaluate Annaletta with regard to object relatedness as it is usually conceived. After testing the psychiatrist and reassuring herself that he was not dangerous, she treated him in a quite impersonal way, as if he were no different from the toys with which she was busily playing. She seemed to regard him as an automaton, an object which might (or might not) help her or provide for her needs, but which had no interest for her in terms of what are generally thought of as peculiarly "human" qualities. On the other hand, she did not avoid the doctor and did not seem to regard him as *less* valuable or interesting than the toys, as some autistic children do.

At the time of our study, no definite diagnosis was made, although she was descriptively a hedonistic child with a very low frustration tolerance and marked distortion of human object relations. Brain damage was considered unlikely, in view of her extraordinary physical agility and dexterity. She entered the children's therapy group, which had been in operation for nearly five months. Mrs. A. was seen individually by a psychiatric resident, since it was felt that she would not fit well into the mothers' group.

Therapy

Annaletta's initial behavior in the group seemed the result of intense anxiety. She screamed, put her hands to her ears, and kept saying, "Goddamn, Goddamn," in a tense, worried voice. She tore off all her clothes and pranced around exhibitionistically. She struck at the other children vigorously and indiscriminately. She climbed upon the window-sill, table, and chairs, and leaped down onto the floor, laughing and muttering gibberish, in a manner more reminiscent of a monkey than a child. At no time did she lose control of her body and she was adept at getting away from the other children when they attacked her. She called all the adults "Marley" and demanded constant attention from them. She wanted to be danced with, swung, or caught, but whenever she jumped into an adult's arms, she would hit, bite, or scratch him, or pull his hair. She seemed afraid of the other children and angry at the therapists for not protecting her from them.

The other children would not tolerate her aggressive behavior and ganged up on her. When she took off her clothes, they hit her, kicked her, and grabbed at her genitals. Whenever the group attacked her, she had violent tantrums, consisting of putting her hands over her ears, shaking her entire body, and screaming "Goddamn." If she were ignored, this would soon subside (Mrs. A. described many similar behavior patterns, both in the home and in public; she insisted that these were "seizures," no different from those for which anticonvulsant medication had been prescribed.) She demanded the attention of the female therapists at all times, and as long as she got it, seemed quite content. However, when she did not get her full attention, she would collect a large amount of saliva in her mouth, push it outward with her tongue, and ultimately spit on the floor. When she jumped and banged into therapists, she would then flash a big, toothy smile, as if to show she was not angry, or to forestall retaliation from the adult. She grabbed at the food and seemingly could not get enough; she took only milk and would not eat the cookies. She often urinated and defecated on the floor, looked anxious, and then attempted to gain forgiveness by "affectionate" behavior towards the therapist. She often masturbated in a frantic, compulsive manner.

Subsequent Course of Therapy

After a time, Annaletta stopped attacking the other children and began playing with them, albeit quite warily. She enjoyed the dances, ring-around-a-rosy, and playing catch. Of the musical instruments, she strongly preferred the drum, which she played with accurate sense of rhythm. At our suggestion, mother dressed her in feminine attire (instead of her usual faded slacks), and the therapists praised her for her appearance. She seemed to become proud of her femininity, and her exhibitionistic behavior lessened markedly.

When crayons were used, she grabbed and hoarded all she could, clutching them tightly in her lap, and became upset if they were taken from her. She was chiefly interested in peeling the paper off the crayons, and in her actual attempts to use them produced only scribbles. Later she began making more recognizably representational drawings which she commented on enthusiastically in her unfathomable jargon. She drew small egg-like things, joined by lines, using mostly black, occasionally red or yellow. When it was time to tidy up the room after this activity, she gathered up a handful of crayons and made a big production of giving them to the therapist. She invariably withheld one crayon, which had to be coaxed from her. She was reluctant to hand crayons or other toys to another child.

When the Tinker Toys were brought into the therapy room, Annaletta seized the box and seemed intent on taking all the pieces for herself, especially the round ones. She held these to her abdomen, retired to a corner of the room, and arranged them in rows or in solid patterns like a pavement. If another child came near, she scattered the toys about wildly, as if to indicate, "If I can't have them, no one else shall." She then gathered up the pieces in her skirt, clutched them tightly to her tummy, sought the female therapist, and handed them to her one by one, then stood back expectantly. When nothing happened, she then searched the therapist's pockets. We later learned that mother always rewarded her with candy whenever she was willing to relinquish an object.

In deciding whether to retain or relinquish, Annaletta seemed to weigh all objects (both things and persons) in terms of possible net loss to herself. This was true of such things as feces, saliva, and urine; food, crayons, toys; and interactions with children. We felt that this behavior indicated her intense attachment to physical objects and her strong conflict over possessing them and letting them go. The conflict seemed to center about the alternatives of physical depletion if she relinquished her objects and loss of love if she retained them. She chose to give up the objects, thereby gaining love, but this exchange seemed a difficult choice, for she always displayed signs of great anxiety in the process.

Dynamic Interaction of Family

An absent father, a disturbed mother barely able to maintain an independent adjustment, and marginal financial means are poor raw materials for an infant to use in developing adequate reality orientation, useful object relationships, and coherent feelings of personal identity. But this was the situation in which Annaletta began her life. While her husband was in the home, providing some emotional and financial support, Mrs. A. remained marginally adjusted. When he was sent to prison, she was unable to maintain this adjustment and became involved in the difficulties which resulted in Annaletta's illegitimate birth. Mrs. A. turned for help to the Welfare Department, who gave her financial assistance and sought to remove the other children from the home because she was too helplessly disorganized to cope with them. The DPW thus unintentionally assumed for Mrs. A. the role of a powerful parent who feeds and protects only the "good" compliant child and frustrates or deprives a "bad" one. Because of her strong dependency and general lack of competence, Mrs. A. could not do without the DPW's help, but her hedonism or lack of coherent organization made it impossible for her to fulfill the DPW's conditions for supplying her needs. We postulated that she found a solution to this dilemma by defining Annaletta as "bad" and herself as the innocent victim of a situation which she dutifully strove to alter, under the benevolent guidance of external authority. Annaletta thus became a specialized extension of Mrs. A. The "bad self" was converted to the "bad child," and her internal struggle to control "badness" was externalized. We also postulated that this solution worked only so long as the child was physically dependent on the mother and unable to separate from her. As Annaletta matured physically, and was increasingly able to separate from mother, the latter's anxiety mounted.

This peculiar form of symbiosis was re-enacted by both mother and child in therapy. Mrs. A. presented herself as a distraught mother unable to control a bad child. She meticulously refrained from overt criticism of her social workers, the Welfare Department, our Clinic, and her individual therapist. She focused on Annaletta's behavior, sought advice on how to control the child, and used her as a lever by which to manipulate social workers and therapists into giving her tangible, concrete assistance, such as money for transportation. When these wishes were frustrated she became intensely angry (probably interpreting refusal as rejection), and this threatened her tenuous control of the rage (badness) which she remained unable to verbalize, despite repeated interpretations. At this juncture, she would find "realistic" reasons for not keeping appointments for two or three sessions. On her return, she would describe how well the child had been until a few days previously, at which time the "bad behavior" had recurred. It was our feeling that mother could not permit her rage at therapist, social workers, and DPW to be expressed except by making use of Annaletta's behavior. When Annaletta's behavior coincided with mother's own feelings of rage and "badness," she was quite tolerable to Mrs. A., and became intolerable only when the disturbance progressed unchecked, or when mother's need for external support reasserted itself. These symbiotic operations seemed to be "security measures" which mother used to maintain her identity, and thus they give clues to the peculiar nature of her object relationships. We noticed early that Mrs. A. tried to manipulate people, and was very good at doing so. When frustrated by people, she would become angry enough to suffer some loss of identity, then retreat from them. She would then later re-emerge as the harried mother and gradually resume her manipulative operations, using Annaletta as an "implement" whereby she could make other people move.

We speculate that Mrs. A. uses manipulation as her chief mode of relating to other people, and at the same time as the principal means of maintaining her own identity. In a two-person system manipulation not only serves to measure and control the distance to "the other," but also to define "the self." In fact, her identity operations and object relationships are so closely intertwined as to be practically identical. Although we do not have positive proof of it, it seems likely that Mrs. A., prior to her symbiotic relationship with her daughter, operated as the junior member of a symbiotic relationship with her mother, and that she has never known other means of defining "self" and "other" except by manipulation. We have speculated that Mrs. A. operated in a symbiotic-manipulative relationship with her first husband, from which he escaped by divorce. A rapid marriage to a second husband recapitulated the situation and terminated when the second husband went to prison. Her needs to define herself via the symbiotic-manipulative relationship resulted in her illegitimate pregnancy, followed by the actions of the DPW in removing her children from the home. It was in this sequence of events and their consequences that Mrs. A. became the senior partner in a symbiotic-manipulative relationship with Annaletta. This relationship with Annaletta represents the safest and most acceptable situation possible for her, and one can see how threatening it might be to Mrs. A. for Annaletta to be "cured."

Annaletta was similarly accustomed to relationships involving control and manipulation of people and things. The group situation quickly disrupted this compulsive, perseverative mode of operation. She responded with panicky, psychotic behavior, including many patterns in which she would race wildly around, then approach the therapist in a placatory manner, as if to re-establish the manipulative interaction which she was accustomed to. Once reassured that her behavior could be accepted, she became less frantic and settled down to a search for identity among inanimate objects which she could manipulate and hoard. We accepted the hoarding temporarily, but in the end she was always forced to relinquish the objects, but without the anger or retaliation she seemed to expect. She repeatedly played out the theme of possessing and giving up objects, found that hoarding was not profitable and that letting go resulted in no actual loss. She then began turning to people as objects and sources of identity (something her disturbed mother was ill-equipped to provide). At the end of two years she had fairly stable object relationships and was using words for purposes of communication. Our early formal identification of Annaletta as a girl (and therefore a definite person) seems to have materially assisted her individuation.

It is difficult to label Annaletta diagnostically. When are alienation from reality and disturbances of self-identity severe enough to call them "psychotic"? Certainly both these factors were present in Annaletta, but not to the degree found in the other four children in the group. Certainly a symbiotic relationship of pathological proportions existed between Annaletta and her mother, but in quite a different way from the other families. Mrs. A. is overtly sick, yet in some ways she is less complicatedly tangled than the other mothers. Though her ego is fragile, it is not encumbered with complex intellectualizations, denial, and reversal, as in the other mothers. She is probably a good deal more consistent than they are in their attitudes towards their children. Obviously some psychotic children have better prognosis than others, and Annaletta's prognosis seems better.

As diagnoses, "pseudo-psychosis" [8] and "borderline state" [9] are misleading, because a psychosis actually does exist. In spite of the seeming ambiguity of the term, "benign psychosis" [10] is perhaps the best way to categorize Annaletta's illness. One member of our group suggested that Annaletta's illness be called a "psychotic situational reaction" inasmuch as it would be impossible to behave in a manner other than psychotic in her environment. Her prognosis may be better because she is psychotic under maximal situational stress, while the other children are psychotic under lesser stresses. Also, she is not withdrawn: she relates to people in a peculiar way, but there is no doubt she is interested and has a lot of "fight." The question of underlying diffuse brain damage remains unanswered, but there is no clear evidence that it exists.

8. B. Rank and S. Kaplan (1951), A case of pseudo-schizophrenia in a child, *American Journal of Orthopsychiatry,* 21:155–181.

9. R. P. Knight (1953), Borderline states, *Bulletin of the Menninger Clinic,* 17:1–12.

10. M. S. Mahler, J. R. Ross, Jr., and Z. De Fries (1949), Clinical studies of benign and malignant cases of childhood psychosis (schizophrenia-like), *American Journal of Orthopsychiatry,* 19:295–305.

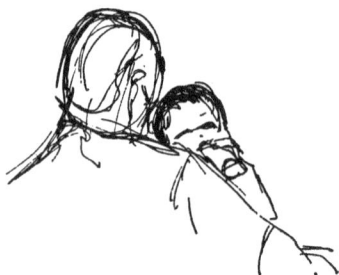

III · The Children's Group:

First Two Years

In this section we shall describe the facilities in which the group therapy was conducted, the interaction between therapist and children, and the vicissitudes of certain drives and behavior patterns. The focus will be on anxiety and aggression, sexuality, excretory activity, attitudes toward food and eating, play activity, and speech.

The children were seen in a room 14 by 20 feet in size. Although exact dimensions are immaterial, the over-all size of the room seems to be important: the room is large enough or long enough to permit momentary withdrawal from the group, but not so large that completely effective withdrawal is possible Our room has one door, which is not locked, but difficult for a child to open because of a husky doorcloser. At the other end of the room is a window at the level of the ground outside, its sill high enough to require strenuous climbing to reach; it was always kept closed, because of the air conditioning. A large mirror covers most of one long wall of the room, and behind it is the observation room; the fourth wall is blank.

The walls are painted a speckled blue and gray. We made the walls as free as possible of all knobs, wires, gadgets, or other hazardous or bothersome protrusions; however, the light-switches can be reached by the children. At first the only article of furniture was a table with a phonograph on it. During the third year, when the children were relating to each other much better, we provided chairs and tables as part of the formal school structure and to allow the group to develop "table manners" while eating. All extraneous objects such as lamps, papers, ash trays, hats and coats are kept outside the room. The original set of play equipment included two rubber balls the size of basketballs, an inflated clown four feet tall (the kind that bobs up when you knock it down), several stuffed animals, and a dozen 1½-inch sponge blocks. The first phonograph records we used were children's stories, but we soon learned that the children disliked these. When we substituted records with catchy, strongly rhythmic tunes, with or without words, they were obviously pleased and seemed calmer and less aggressive. Loud marching tunes, to which the therapists beat time with hands or feet, were most effective in alleviating group tensions and anxieties.

Our observations of autism in psychotic children had led us to postulate that it is a defensive attitude used to preserve infantile omnipotence. Thus, when autistic, the child omnipotently controls the "distance" in the symbiosis, preventing engulfment of self or of mother, and similarly preventing loss or separation of self from mother. Early in group therapy, the autistic defense fails, either due to the enhanced anxiety resulting from the new and unfamiliar situation, or because of the active penetration of the defense by the behavior of the other children in the group. The most immediate and urgent problem facing the therapist was dealing with the resulting panic. The small size of the room prevented physical isolation, and the actively aggressive behavior of two of the children made psychic withdrawal impossible; panic occurred when physical reality could no longer be handled by autistic denial.

Mike and Walter attempted to maintain their autistic defenses, while Annaletta became aggressively exhibitionistic and Bob was provocatively aggressive. Tina seemed more like a child with primary autism who had never experienced symbiosis. The therapists soon became involved in efforts to restrain the aggressive children and protect the withdrawn ones. The children manifested their panic by diffuse, rage-like, self-destructive behavior, falling to the floor, biting hands and arms, and banging head and arms on the floor. We intervened by holding the child, attempting to comfort him by reassurances and soothing gestures. This was rarely successful, and so we tried promoting regression, by holding the child like a nursing infant and offered a baby bottle of milk. The children varied in their acceptance of regression, but the permissive, even seductive, attitude of the therapists enabled the panicky child to accept this method of coping with the disintegrative threat. The children's panic reactions provoked much anxiety in the therapists, but once convinced of the effectiveness of this technique, they developed a sense of security which was evidently transmitted to the children. Some of the children seemed intolerant of the closeness involved in being held and this presented difficulties. Gentle, firm techniques of restraint which avoided face-to-face closeness, but left the child effectively under the physical control of the therapist, were most effective. The therapist sat behind the child, wrapped his legs around the child's, crossed the child's arms in front of him and held the wrists firmly (as in a straitjacket), and, if necessary, immobilized the child's head with his chin to keep the child from banging his head against the therapist's chest. A child can be held in this position for long periods of time without much discomfort to either party, and the child will ultimately respond by stopping the self-destructive behavior. We also learned that the mirror could be of great value in controlling panic. We took the child to the mirror, touched and named him and the various parts of his body. Each person in the room was also named and pointed out in the mirror. We often noted that when anxiety threatened to overwhelm a child, he would get as close to the mirror as possible, as though to correlate touch and sight, and thus maintain identity.

Aggression

Once we had effectively controlled the rage-like behavior, subsequent interaction of the child and the therapeutic environment led to aggressive behavior directed diffusely outward, not toward any particular object. At one point, four of the children were behaving in this way, and it was necessary to have three therapists in the room at once in order to control the situation. Tina was not involved in this, and our task was to protect her from the aggression of the others, as she responded only with apparent puzzlement when attacked. Under the constant application of firm but gentle physical restraint, the aggressivity became less diffuse, more goal-directed, and eventually was mostly confined to retaliation: the children would "gang up" defensively against a child who attacked aggressively. Each child in turn, except Tina, tried being provocative or aggressive and was met with the mutually protective opposition of the rest of the group. Thus each child developed respect for the restraining and retaliatory power of the group, and provocative behavior of this sort practically disappeared. The provocation was not always deliberate in nature, but could be viewed simply as the discharge of aggressive but unhostile impulses; at times it seemed to be a way of differentiating self from not-self or from inanimate objects; at other times it was probably a primitive way of making contact with another child. Sometimes it was obviously open hostility toward a child misidentified as a hated sibling.

When Annaletta entered the group during the fifth month

of therapy, the group's anxiety was intensified, and it seemed as though the boys were intent on destroying her or forcibly ejecting her from the group. She herself was very anxious and discharged her tension in exhibitionistically aggressive behavior. Her speed and dexterity foiled the boys' efforts to demolish her, and her hyperactive behavior also prevented them from ignoring her. As a result, the group was exceedingly tense for nearly six weeks, but we feel that she also acted as an important catalyst for group formation. Tina was very intrigued by Annaletta and mimicked her in every activity except removing her clothing. A typical pattern of Annaletta's was to enter the room in a state of marked anxiety, immediately disrobing and jumping about the room in an effort to deal with the anxiety through violent physical activity. She seemed to be hungry for object relationships, but feared closeness. She aggressively approached each child in the group, momentarily overwhelmed him, then dashed off to another child or to an adult. Her gibberish and gestures, along with her nudity, made the other children anxious too; in an effort to reduce their own anxieties, the children attacked and attempted to subdue her, but were baffled by her agility. Gradually she became more tolerant of contact with the adults and other children, and the general tension of the group subsided. Thus her provocative behavior (as in the previous case of the other children's provocative behavior) promoted group formation, and the more passive children found themselves joining forces in order to deal with her bewildering aggression.

After eight months of therapy (three months for Annaletta) the children's aggressive behavior was largely limited to situations involving competition for an adult's attention, analogous to sibling rivalry. The jealous child would attack both the rival and the adult who was supplying the attention. Later, the jealous attack was limited to the child, and not always in the immediate situation, but delayed and executed in another situation. Group interpretations of fear, anger, and jealousy of one another, and of real siblings, were repeated many times. After a year of therapy, aggression was more nearly like that of normal children, mostly involving property rights, although jealousy situations were still frequent.

When the four new children (Melvin, Ralph, Carol, and Kate) were added during the thirteenth month, we anticipated a recrudescence of the aggression, but were surprised when the children of the original group seemed to identify with the therapists and actually assisted in quieting the panic of the new ones. It seemed to us that the new children's panic threatened the original group members and perhaps evoked memories of their own panic states of the past. Rather than trying to annihilate the inciting ones, they attempted to alleviate the panic by techniques which had worked with them. Thus, we saw Mike lead Ralph to the mirror, gently touch various parts of his body while naming them and naming the other members of the group. At various times, members of the original group were seen feeding milk to the new children with the baby bottles or leading an anxious child to the therapist for comforting. However, when a child cried in a tantrum, he was attacked. When Melvin joined the group he ignored everyone and lay on the floor rolling his head from side to side, making loud moaning sounds. The children watched his performance curiously and gradually came closer to him. If one of them touched him, he jumped up, dashed to another spot, and resumed his posture and behavior. The children then made a game of straddling Melvin without touching him. When this had been done many times, Melvin was seen to clutch Walter by the knees as if to hold him, but at the same time kicking him away, thus dramatically demonstrating his ambivalence about closeness. But the children persisted in the game, and soon Melvin gave up this activity except in situations where he was fairly severely frustrated. Walter imitated Melvin's behavior several times, and Melvin broke out with genuine laughter at this.

The generally more stable situation allowed Ralph to withdraw more than had been possible with the original group, and he was later able to enter into group activity without being attacked, probably because he was not particularly aggressive or provocative. Melvin frequently attacked Tina and Carol, but not Annaletta. Bob seemed to identify with the girls in the situation and would retaliate against Melvin on behalf of the girls. Walter and Bob frequently wrestled and chased one another, which frightened Carol. She often cried in this situation and then would be the target for an attack by Mike. Walter was consistently a problem in the group in that he acted on all aggressive impulses (whether hostile or unhostile) with little evidence of internal control. The children would often gang up on him for this behavior, but this only seemed to enhance his aggressivity and eventuated in considerable withdrawal by most of the other children. In these scuffles, there were marked contrasts in behavior and affect between Walter and the others. When attacked, Bob became enraged and/or terrified; he would turn red in the face, scream, and dash to the mirror, where he made faces at himself. Mike turned on Walter and kicked or bit him methodically. Melvin sought protection by an adult. The girls would cry and scream. If, on the other hand, one or more children attacked Walter, he would laughingly respond as though it were a game, becoming very aggressive, without regard to dangers to others or himself. When it came to property rights or space rights, the children were disinclined to permit Walter to get away with his confiscatory attitudes and would often gang up on him. Once convinced that he could not get away with this behavior, he confined himself to his own domain. A type of "pecking order" developed in the group, with Walter at the top and Kate at the bottom. Displacement to inanimate objects was also frequent.

To summarize, the anxiety produced in the group by the physical closeness of the children and the adults resulted in penetration and disruption of the autistic defenses of these children. The inability to further ignore and deny the reality situation produced overwhelming panic in each child, manifested by diffuse, rage-like disintegrative and self-destructive activity. In this situation the therapist must be very active in providing opportunities for regression and for strong external support and restraint for the child. Such activity on the part of the therapist assists the child to cope with the psychotic anxiety and to discharge tension through outwardly directed aggressive behavior. When controls are consistently applied, along with verbalized reassurances of protection, the controls become internalized to a remarkable degree. It is important to recognize that the "reassurance" is not simply, "Everything is going to be all right," but rather involves a factual, reassuring statement to the effect, "Dr. Speers *can* control Bob." Group formation then becomes a reality, and each child learns respect for the retaliatory powers of the group. The group becomes a "safe" alternative to autism and its integrity is essential to its members.

The children were disturbed by the intrusion of new children or adults in the group and by the absence of any of the usual participants: When Annaletta was not there, Bob wondered if she were dead, and was anxious until the therapist provided an explanation of her absence. Within the therapeutic group there developed a "group ego" with constantly improving abilities for reality testing and object relatedness. It is our belief that separation-individuation processes (which normally occur in the context of a normal mother-child symbiosis) took place in the context of a relatively healthy symbiosis between the group and the individual children.

It was also evident that the group therapy experiences were carried over into other group situations as well as the home environment. By the end of the second year, four of the five original children had been in ordinary kindergartens in their home towns. This went on for a period of months without undue strain on teachers or classmates. Walter's uninhibited but unhostile aggression presented a problem both in the group and outside, but this was primarily the result of his parents' inability to place realistic limits on his behavior.

Excretory Activity

Of the original five children, only Bob was completely toilet trained. Walter and Annaletta used the toilet, but did so only out of fear of mother. Mike used defecation as a way of defying his mother, and in the group situation, as a means of implementing his autistic withdrawal by keeping others at a distance. Tina seemed oblivious of the excretory process. When Annaletta entered the group, she discharged much of her anxiety in excretory exhibitionism and often defecated and urinated on the floor. This seemed to focus the attention of the group on excretory functions, and all became very much aware of this activity. Mike and Bob watched Annaletta avidly but anxiously and mimicked her. Walter was also obviously anxious; he could not look directly, but stole sidelong glances at Annaletta's performance. He did start soiling himself at home, and when his mother put him back in diapers, he seemed quite confused. Tina watched with interest and made attempts to play with the excreta of the others, but seemed unaware of her own capacities. We got mother to put only one diaper on her, instead of two, after which she became acquainted with her own excretory capabilities and soon mimicked Annaletta's behavior. Next, we offered to take the children to the toilet, and this produced a remarkable effect: It afforded the children a chance to get away from the tension and anxiety of the group situation as well as getting individual attention from the female therapist. Thus two of the strongest motivations were combined, and this is probably why toilet training actually took place. Once in the bathroom, the children were permitted a moderate amount of exhibitionism, fecal play, smearing, and the right to flush the toilet and observe the swirling contents disappear. It was quite evident from the children's facial expressions that the feces were proudly offered as a "gift," and the therapists responded warmly, with appropriate enthusiasm. It soon became unacceptable to excrete in the group therapy room, and violations were met by physical attacks. Toilet training had not been a specific goal of our treatment program, but quite obviously the moves we made to handle the situation were effective in producing actual training as a sort of "free" by-product.

The condition of being trained carried over to the home situation, and further difficulty was reported only by Mike's mother, who related that he continued to deposit feces in odd places about the house in defiance of her. Once she had discussed some memories of her wishes to soil herself in defiance of her own mother's strict rules about cleanliness, Mike's behavior in this regard ceased.

Thus all the children became toilet trained by, or through, the following process: First, they actually became aware of the act of excretion; a reasonable amount of play and exhibitionism was permitted; a reward was offered for excretory control (escape from the group and sole possession of the female therapist); they were permitted to smear, and their compliantly produced "gifts" were praised; finally, group pressure disapproving excretory misbehavior rendered the training complete within the group formation. At home, the maternal attitude toward excretory functions sometimes had to be altered before training was complete in the usual sense.

When the four new children were added, we anticipated regression in toilet activity, but this did not occur. However, we did not achieve the same kind of training results with the new children as we had with the original group. We had placed a potty chair in the group room but only the two girls would use it as a toilet; the boys used it for urination, but not for defecation. The new children were curious about the potty chair, but showed little interest or curiosity about excretory acts. Carol seemed quite distressed by the potty and while she made gestures toward it, such as pulling down her panties and sitting on it, refused to use it as a toilet. Melvin delighted in turning it over once it had been used. Ralph and Kate ignored it. We speculated that the original group's attitude towards excretory activity was like pressure from the outside to the new children, rather than something stemming from a group ego, which is more like inside pressure. The new children were not yet integrated into the group, hence not participants in the group ego.

When we moved into a new therapy room containing a sink and an adjoining lavatory, the children showed renewed interest in toilet play. The interest, however, was not concentrated on excretion or excreta, but more on the disappearance of material when the toilet was flushed. This was pronounced with Tina, Mike, and Walter but minimal with Annaletta and Bob. Melvin spent a good deal of time sitting on the toilet, but rarely produced anything. Ralph and Kate paid no attention to it, but soiled themselves at will. Carol used the toilet to allay her fears of soiling herself when she got angry; she would go through all the motions of warning us non-verbally, (and verbally saying, "Go to bathroom"), but once she was in the bathroom, she did nothing further. (We later learned that this was a replication of a recurrent situation at home whereby she controlled her parents by claiming she had to go to the bathroom and then got them upset by tearfully refusing to do anything.) The "old" children used the toilet in the development of realistic ideas about objects, and they verbalized numerous concerns about "holes" and "gone away." This may have been initially related to their wishes to get rid of the new children in the group and their siblings at home. It was also in this context that the group verbalized their ideas about the connection between ingested food and eventual excretory products. Thus a number of fears, anxieties, and reality-testing problems were worked through in the toilet situation.

Here is a typical behavior sequence: The group is crayoning, and Walter, jealous of Mike's productions, manages to scribble and ruin Mike's drawing. Mike becomes enraged and hits at Walter, who laughingly dashes out of Mike's reach. Mike then turns over a chair in anger, tears off a bit of drawing paper, and runs to the bathroom, where he joyfully throws it into the bowl and flushes the toilet. As he watches the paper swirl out of sight, he becomes anxious and grabs at it. He is unable to reach it in time and has a look of anxiety on his face. Quickly he rushes out of the bathroom into the playroom. The moment he sees Walter, the look of anxiety fades and he returns to his drawing.

Another sequence: Walter had been referred to as "King Walter" because of his imperious, arrogant attitude toward everything in the room. He seemed to resent the implication of this title and on one occasion tore paper into little bits, threw them into the toilet, and designated them as "Dr. Speers." Then he happily flushed the toilet and ecstatically announced, "Now, King Walter."

There was definite correlation between the degree of toilet training and the ability to use messy play materials such as finger paint, clay, dough, and mud pies. Only after toilet training was complete did the children make wholehearted use of such materials. The untrained children (Ralph and Melvin) continued to use them reluctantly. Kate seemed unable to distinguish her feces from the play material; for instance, she was often observed to reach into her pants for feces during sessions with the finger paint.

Sexuality

Early in therapy, the only activity that could be called sexual was when Tina reached into the boys' pants trying to find the penis. Annaletta was the catalyst for more vigorous sexual behavior, primarily exhibitionism, but also acting out concerns about the integrity of the penis and the differences between boys and girls.

As soon as Annaletta entered the room, she would begin taking off her clothes and would dance around in such a way as to attract attention, dancing in front of people and looking intently at their faces as if to gauge their response, and seemingly forcing the attention of the therapists to her activity, a kind of "fascination." Bob would immediately respond by disrobing too. Mike watched intently but anxiously. Walter did not seem anxious but watched the performance with interest. Tina imitated the affective expressions of the others and made efforts to remove her own clothing. Mike closely inspected Annaletta's genitals, then ran to the mirror to look into his mouth, then requested that all the adults open their mouths for inspection. He ecstatically announced "two penises" (presumably the second was the uvula) and grabbing at his genitals, danced about excitedly. He told his parents, "Everyone in the room has a penis but Annaletta." Annaletta's exhibitionism became more and more provocative, and it seemed as though she were using her entire body as a phallus. Walter and Mike's response seemed to be aimed at proving that she did not have a penis. They attacked her viciously and grabbed at her genitals. We assisted her in abandoning this phallic role by pointing out and complimenting her on her feminine features, such as her hair, and encouraged her mother to dress her as a girl. Ultimately she became proud of her femininity and gave up the phallic exhibitionism. Bob attempted to continue his exhibitionistic behavior even though Annaletta had altered hers, and this led to his also being attacked by the rest of the group. They focused primarily on his penis and seemed bent on pulling it off. Bob often expressed the wish to "be a girl like sister"; the other children may have been attacking him to check on the chances of such a possibility, or because the idea threatened them. At any rate, the group pressures forced Bob to remain clothed. During this phase, the therapists made statements about the differences between the boys and girls and the permanency of such differences. When Tina later began to urinate and defecate exhibitionistically, the boys once again became quite curious, but did no more than look. Mike, however, was determined to demonstrate the anatomic identity of the two sexes. He did this by ignoring the genitals and focusing on the anus. "Tina has an anus, Mike has an anus, everybody has an anus," he proudly announced. He subsequently named all the parts of the body that are alike, carefully avoiding mentioning the penis. He often sang, "Tina has an anus," over and over as if to relieve anxiety. He frequently clutched his genitals, or pulled out the waistband of his trousers to take a look at them. He often had erections and made numerous attempts to rub against the female workers and to fondle their breasts. Whenever Mike could not avoid seeing Tina's genitals, he closed his eyes, ran to the male therapist, and buried his head in his lap, crying. The therapist responded sympathetically, interpreting Mike's fear of losing his penis.

Bob and Walter similarly had frequent erections and made similar attempts to loll on the female therapists. The therapist gently but firmly restrained this activity, commenting that it had to do with the child's fear about his penis both in the therapy situation and at home. Overt genital masturbation was rare in the boys but common in the girls. In Tina the pattern was analogous to her previous behavior of mouthing objects and playing with the boys' penises, in that she used it both as an attention-getting device and a compulsive activity for the release of tension. Group pressure, in the form of physical interference, made Tina stop her overt masturbatory behavior.

When the four new children were added, there was a mild recurrence of interest in anatomy; however, these interests were now verbalized, not acted out. Each child was designated as boy or girl by each member of the "old" group and once the distinction was confirmed by the therapists, there was little further interest. The other children watched with interest as Bob played out his intense anxieties about sexual differences with the dolls, and quite often one of them would imitate this, putting himself in the principal role. There was a great deal of concern about bodily integrity, what people are made of and what would happen if one child were to hurt another child. Anatomical differences seemed very important to Carol, and we gained the impression that she was denying her lack of a penis. When one of the male children exhibited his penis, Carol became very upset, clutched her own genitals, and dashed for the toilet. Ralph, Melvin, and Kate seemed quite unconcerned about these differences and paid little attention to such behavior. Melvin, however, was more prone to attack females than males. Kate liked to play with Carol's foot in a way that many of us interpreted as interest in a penis. When Carol became anxious she grabbed at the genitals of the male children and therapists, but this was done in such a manner as to make it appear almost accidental, and so there was little retaliation against her by the boys.

We dealt with the children's fantasies about sexual matters by encouraging them to clarify the content by detailed verbalization, and then we attempted to correct the distortion in the fantasies by asserting the facts. Interspersed with the numerous questions about sexual anatomic differences were statements and questions regarding the whereabouts of mother, father, an absent child, or a child's mother who was absent from the group. Likewise, there was both verbal and nonverbal designation of the male therapists as father, the female therapists as mother, and other personnel as teacher, uncle, or aunt.

It thus became apparent to us that the children were busily engaged in comparing notes about similarities and differences and that this was furthering separation-individuation. It seemed important that we recognize this progression of fantasy material as a step in self-definition. The children started this process with concern over body parts and name differences, followed by the boy-girl distinction. They then branched out to external possessions: mothers, fathers, etc., and again compared notes. It was as if each child could conceptualize the idea "I am a person like you, because by a remarkable coincidence it turns out that both of us have mothers." It of course turns out that all the children have this in common, and this was another defining feature of the abstract concept of "a person" which was forming in the group. This spread to other relatives in common, like fathers and uncles and aunts, and this furthered the line of self-definition. It was as though the children discovered that points in common are invariant marks of humanity, whereas points of difference are marks of individuality, separateness, and uniqueness.

Food

The initial extreme of refusing or gluttonously devouring the refreshments gradually changed, with recognition that the food was being offered for their pleasure and comfort without implications of reward or punishment. The early regressive attitudes were accepted and indulged as much as possible, in order to promote corrective emotional experiences regarding food was being offered for their pleasure and comfort with food, allowing Walter to have food fads, not bribing Mike, and undoing the implications of reward and punishment with Annaletta. Bob was allowed to regress to sucking, after which he voluntarily gave this up and progressed to more mature attitudes.

When the new children were added to the group, regressive feeding behavior on their part was similarly permitted both by the therapists and the original group of children. Gradually the cookies-and-milk time became an event which the children greatly enjoyed, and the group's hustle and bustle to clean things up was evidence of their pleasurable anticipation. We permitted any behavior with food except purposely throwing it at another child. From this restraint and from group pressures, a "table morality" evolved which is quite comparable to that of a group of normal children. Ultimately table conversation occurred, with exchange of direct questions and answers among the children. They also indicated their pleasure in the meal-time situation by imitating one another, followed by laughter. For instance, if a child grunted in asking for more milk, another child would imitate this behavior, and then the entire group would laugh. The children also verbalized fantasies about food, where it goes in and how it comes out.

Play

Play activity changed considerably during the therapy, both from the standpoint of materials we provided and how the children responded. At first the children used toys as objects to relate to in an autistic way, or as aggressive weapons to drive away intrusive representatives of reality. We soon learned that any hard object would be used as a weapon, so that we had to exclude such things as wooden blocks, sticks, toy automobiles, and dolls. If there were too many items, the children seemed confused and could not settle down to one toy without being distracted by the impulse to explore the others. At the height of the aggressive period (fourth to seventh month) we did without toys altogether, but instead kept the music going constantly and encouraged the children to clap hands and stomp feet together as a group, in order to channel their intense destructive energy into a bearable form. We felt that the music was effective in this situation.

We designated the inflated plastic clown as something which the children could aggress against, and the therapists often demonstrated this, without many takers. However, the children were willing to kick the walls instead of people, and so we reinforced this as a way for them to deal acceptably with hostile feelings. The children threw toys as offensive weapons and as symbols of their wish to throw the other children out. When this happened, we removed the toys and offered active group games. The children seemed to enjoy the "all fall down" part of ring-around-a-rosy a great deal and repeated it many, many times. At such times, individuals would also pair off and play running and chasing games, which seemed to alleviate tension nicely. This primarily involved Bob, Walter, and Annaletta, while Tina tried to imitate their activity and affect. Her own affect was really quite flat, and she seemed to want to duplicate the facial expressions of enjoyment and excitement which the others exhibited and the noises that they made.

Mike steadfastly refused to enter into this sort of play, but later was seen to be operating on the fringes of the ring-around-a-rosy games, far enough away to remain separate from the group. This resembled the type of parallel play which is seen in two- and three-year-old nursery school children, in which they do the same thing alongside one another but do not interact or influence each other's activities significantly. If taken by the hand, Mike would enter the group for a few moments only. Then we noticed the children were reaching their hands out to one another in order to form a circle for the game. They communicated non-verbally to the adults their desires to be danced with, lifted, swung, raised up to the ceiling, chased, caught, and tickled. The therapists responded to these group requests with considerable enthusiasm. This led to noticeable sibling rivalry and gave us an idea of how intense was the desire for an exclusive one-to-one relationship. However, after we interpreted their feelings on this score, they seemed fairly willing to wait and take turns. Once we had a gas-balloon on the ceiling, whose string was too short for the children to reach. They would be lifted up to grab at the balloon, then set down to release the balloon again; during the game they formed a line and willingly waited their turns. On another occasion we introduced a chair with wheels into the room, and the children took turns pushing and riding in it:

two would ride, two would push, and one would guide the chair.

When we introduced dolls early in therapy, the children promptly pulled them apart, without any attempt to put them back together again. Similarly they lost interest in hitting the clown, and instead took to deflating it as soon as they entered the room.

A general description of this early "play" activity demonstrates each child's way of avoiding group interactions. Mike managed to find a phonograph record and seemed to pretend that he was the phonograph, twirling around with the record held in his hand until the other children forced him to stop. Walter selected a stuffed animal, and would walk around the room with it tightly clutched to his body, and with thumb in mouth would effectively avoid the group until someone snatched the toy away from him. Tina preferred shoe laces, and would sit and suck on a lace until another child managed to pull it away from her. Annaletta liked to climb monkey-like along the window-sill, the lower frame of the big mirror-window and the table-top, uttering gibberish and then jumping down to the floor with much excitement. Bob always retreated to the female worker and got as close to her as he could, all the time talking baby talk to gain undivided attention. Thus every child tended to relate to one thing or one person in order to avoid contact with the group as a whole, and the anxiety engendered by such contact. Group interaction occurred sporadically and lasted only a few moments, but as time went on, the children gradually increased their tolerance for the group.

Around the ninth month of therapy we felt that the children were ready for structured activities and decided to try the following ones to start off: Blowing soap bubbles, crayoning, Tinker Toys, throwing a ball, ring-around-a-rosy, finger painting, and the percussion band. In order to release tensions at the beginning of the sessions, we always began with one of the more violent activities, such as ring-around-a-rosy, tag, throwing and catching a ball, London Bridge, or follow-the-leader. The phonograph provided a musical background, and we kept it going rather loud. After this, we introduced soapy water and straws. The children sat around a pan of water, dabbled in it, sucked it up in the straws, blew bubbles into the water, slopped it on the floor and each other, and even tried to bathe in it. Gradually, however, imitating the therapists and later each other, the children attempted to blow bubbles in the air, with varying degrees of success. Mike learned quickly and took pleasure in showing off his skill. Walter succeeded accidentally, but would not follow up; he blew into the basin instead, creating a mass of more nearly permanent bubbles. Tina and Bob tried, but blew too hard. Annaletta would not try to make bubbles, but played with the water and straws.

As soon as the children grew restless with the bubble activity, the water, straws, and towels were removed and were replaced by crayoning material. Each child was assigned to a section outlined on a large sheet of brown paper which was placed on the floor, with the crayons dumped in the middle of it. At first Tina and Annaletta wanted to take and hoard all the crayons but gradually we induced them to take only those they needed for drawing. Each child had a favorite color and produced a characteristic stereotyped drawing. Annaletta liked black and always drew circles which she then joined by a myriad of lines. Sometimes she would make a red or yellow circle in the center. Mike liked to draw pumpkins, beach balls, and balloons and preferred orange colors. He would also draw triangles, squares, and trapezoids, which he named. His art work was very skillful. He became angry when forced to stay within his own space on the paper and pouted if another child marked up his allotted space. Tina made circular scrawls and preferred purple. Bob scribbled violently in all directions and had no favorite color. Once he created a multi-colored design and asked that it be cut out so he could take it home. Walter chose orange, green, or yellow, always peeled off the paper covering of the crayon, and then in a vigorous vertical motion made a solid block of color on the paper. Sometimes he did this with circular motions.

As the children became bored with the drawings with crayons, they would indulge in hoarding activities or start throwing the crayons around; at this point the crayons would be removed. The children enjoyed using the paper during the subsequent part of the session, and this was permitted. Bob often used it as a skirt. Tinker Toys were then brought in and dumped in a pile on the floor, and the children all tried to grab as many as they could. Annaletta picked up all the round pieces she could find, and clutching them to her tummy in her skirt, moved away from the group and arranged them in a solid, pavement-like pattern on the floor. If another child approached her, she would mess up the pattern. Later, she gathered and hoarded the straight sticks and offered them one at a time to the female worker. Walter always took the green sticks and a hub, and made a rimless wheel; he then moved away from the group and twirled the wheel, with one thumb in his mouth. Tina early learned to put two or three pieces together; she seemed pleased at this success and would make several of these constructions. Bob usually put several pieces in his mouth and sat around daydreaming, but when given undivided attention by the female worker, he constructed a creditable automobile on several occasions. Mike built fantastic structures to which he gave fanciful names; he said one was a "bathtub," and then related a fantasy of being in a bathtub with mother and his sister, Jeannette. When in a pouting mood, he made nothing. He was rather jealous of Walter's creations and seemed to want to make something better.

The Tinker Toys were then removed and the percussion band brought in. Although for a while they were afraid of the cymbals and drums, the children soon expressed delight when band time arrived. Walter chose the xylophone and with thumb in mouth would hit one note only, but with an attempt at rhythm. Tina selected the triangle, and although at times she preferred to suck the striker, generally followed the rhythm and danced about during this activity. Annaletta and Bob liked the drums and sticks and viciously beat the drum without regard to rhythm, although Annaletta danced, and later drummed, with excellent rhythm. Mike chose the cymbals and marched around like a drum major. A loud marching-band record played during this activity. The children participated with much jumping, dancing, clapping of hands, and banging of instruments.

Later we introduced jigsaw puzzles of various kinds, and these were very popular. Mike and Walter put them together rapidly and accurately. Walter went according to form only, without regard to color or picture content, not even using the borders as normal children do; he showed great frustration when he could not make a piece fit. Mike at the start assembled the pieces by form only but later learned to go by color and content. Both he and Walter commented on what the picture was about, and Mike was able to fantasy a past and future for the picture. Tina attempted to work these puzzles, but with only moderate success, while Bob and Annaletta had no interest in them at all.

When we introduced clay as a play material, several of the children ate it, and there was very little attempt to use it to make things. Finger painting provoked too much anxiety in the children early in therapy, but was later enjoyed (after 18 months of therapy). In addition to playing indoors, we took the children outside when the weather was nice and permitted considerable free play in a large enclosed yard. A plastic wading pool was available and a water hose which when turned on provided seemingly joyful interaction among the children. They used only sparingly a sandbox and sand toys.

Beginning in the ninth month, we began an individual session for each child with the occupational therapist, one hour per week. The content of the two therapeutic situations showed an interesting contrast. In the doll play of the individual sessions the "child" doll was constantly with the "mother" doll, and the fantasies seemed to center on the theme of maintaining a one-to-one relationship with the adult. In the group sessions, the action and fantasies concerned competition and rivalry, perhaps an attempt to establish or regain a one-to-one relationship.

When the children became more proficient in any type of play activity, it seemed expedient to introduce new activities. Eventually it became clear that they were ready for more formal activities such as might prepare them for kindergarten and school. Our plans for this change were interrupted by the entry of the new children into the group, and it was then necessary to repeat much of the play activity that the original group had already mastered in order to bring the new children up to their level. This was effective with Carol, less so with Ralph, and ineffective with Melvin and Kate. We felt that we should not hold back the original group any longer and so we decided to introduce some abstract materials to assist in school readiness. We used form boards with simple geometrical shapes, some involving colors, and some for letters and numbers.

In September, 1961, Walter, Tina, Mike, and Bob were placed in kindergartens near their homes and were able to adjust without much difficulty. It was felt that they had been able to transfer the group-therapy experience to the new group situation, and that remarkably little anxiety had ensued. Annaletta might well have handled such a situation, but her mother was unwilling to let her attend nursery school or kindergarten at that time.

Speech

At the beginning of therapy all the children had quite severe problems of speech and communication. Bob spoke in an infantile singsong voice which was practically unintelligible; this seemed to be an obsessive (or controlling) activity, and was not meant for verbal communication. In content it consisted primarily of demanding phrases which sounded like parental commands. In an exhibitionistic way, Mike frequently uttered isolated words or phrases of which we could make no sense. He would say things like "tubes," "Mama bear," "Papa bear," accompanied by ecstatic gestures and bizarre posturing. Tina made faces and gestures that seemed like mimicry of her mother and uttered grunts and noises, but not formed syllables. Walter was totally silent and expressionless. Annaletta excitedly uttered rapid gibberish, with many gestures and facial grimaces. Her "faces" may have had communicative meaning but the gibberish did not seem to: the only words we could understand were "Goddamn, Goddamn."

We noted changes in speech, once the initial aggressive behavior had come under control. Walter primarily communicated negative feelings; when offered milk, he would grunt, squeal, stamp his foot, and turn his back on the person who offered it. We later heard him utter squeals of delight when playing, and he seemed to be experimenting with making sounds. Later we noted that he was moving his mouth as if to speak, but no words came forth. We tried to convey the attitude that we did not care whether he talked or not, but that he could if he wanted to. When we saw him apparently talking "under his breath," we told him, "You may speak if you wish." He said a few words and seemed delighted. He later communicated his wants with words as well as grunts, gestures, and "faces." If someone asked him a question, he was most reluctant to answer it, but if *he* wanted something, he would use words readily enough. After two years of therapy, Walter's speech was still rather infantile and difficult to understand unless one listened carefully. Although he was very curious and wanted answers to many questions, he tended to use one-syllable words, and only two or three words per message. The indistinctness of his speech may have been partly due to his unwillingness to look at people when talking. With the speech therapist, who consistently urged the children to watch and imitate, Walter displayed keen interest in pronouncing words more correctly and was beginning to lose some of the infantile quality of his speech.

Tina's mimicry of facial and gestural affective expressions gradually extended to mimicry of words and speech, which slowly led to the development of a vocabulary which is, however, considerably smaller than that of a normal child of her age. At first she was more interested in communicating parental-type prohibitions by word and gesture, but extended this to expressions of her own wants. Her speech was clear, but her communications were not always relevant to the actual situation.

We interpreted Annaletta's gibberish to her as expressing her desire to keep our attention, but at the same time to keep us at a distance. We insisted that she speak if she wished a response, and we complimented her speech as it developed. We felt that only as her anxiety decreased was she able to take the time to learn to speak. Her frequent absences were associated with regression, which was most clearly shown in her speech; if she missed more than two sessions, she returned to her original mode of verbal expressions: gibberish.

Mike's speech underwent profound changes. After two years, he often communicated in long, relevant sentences, with correct use of pronouns. There was a rather irritating exhibitionistic quality to his remarks, but we ignored this aspect as long as his communications seemed to relate validly to his feelings or the immediate situation.

By the end of two years, Bob used pronouns correctly, but his voice still retained its infantile singsong quality. He communicated all his concerns, but when we asked for clarification of a statement, he did not seem to understand. His remarks were quite obsessive, but he was well aware of reality.

At first, communication between the children was largely of the non-verbal kind, but they did unmistakably communicate. Later, verbal interchanges were common, especially with Tina, Mike, Bob, and Annaletta, less so with Walter.

There was often a good deal of talk between a child and the adults in the room, particularly questions about the other children, for instance, questions about a child who had been taken to the toilet. There was always great concern over Annaletta's frequent absences and many questions about where she was and when she would return. In this situation, we would clarify their fantasies that they had harmed her and correlate these with fantasies about their own siblings at home, whom they wanted to be rid of. If they anxiously asked questions when another child was crying, we clarified the difference between crying-when-hurt and crying like a hungry, unhappy, angry baby. On the other hand, there was much curiosity about "things" and the names of all objects, colors, and people. The children constantly mimicked one another, which indicated an acute awareness (not necessarily an integrated one) of the group and the individuals who comprised it. But when a child had a tantrum, the other children usually attacked him, and when prevented, they asked questions about "mad" and "bad." We generally interpreted the situation to the children as one in which *they* saw the offender's action as "bad" and angry and wished to eliminate the child in question for fear of losing control of their own angry impulses. On the other hand, laughter became commonplace, and the children seemed to get genuine pleasure from their play.

The introduction of the new children did seem to interrupt the therapeutic progress of the group for a while, but this soon abated and the "old" children's former level of behavior was resumed. We added these four new children to the group (with some misgivings) because they appeared on our doorstep, so to speak, needed treatment, and met our criteria for age and diagnosis. We also wished to enlarge the group somewhat, since during the winter months two or three absent children left us with a very small group indeed. Perhaps the most difficult part of the situation was the narcissistic investment of the therapists in the original group members. We feared that the new children would disturb the level of maturation which the original group members had achieved, and hence had considerable feelings of anxiety and hostility about the new ones. Although we could not be sure that the therapists' discomfort in this situation had much to do with the regression of the "old" group, once these feelings were discussed in the supervisory sessions, the "old" children regained their former level of adjustment.

The correlation of anxiety with speech variation was striking in these children. When Bob was anxious and became infantile in his speech, he referred to himself as "Bob" (instead of "I") and obsessively asked irrelevant questions. Mike exhibitionistically shouted his knowledge and concern about penises when he was anxious, while Ralph became echolalic. A fascinating aspect of this echolalia was the complete difference between his echolalic voice and his "own" voice. The latter was appropriately infantile in tone, and the content appropriate to a child; the echolalia was obvious mimicry of mother in tone quality and content. Carol's voice had some peculiar aspects. Her "accent" might have been related to the fact that her mother is British, but in the mothers' therapy group we noted that the mother's own accent was minimal; it may be different at home and Carol may have been imitating a kind of speech that we never heard. When she was anxious, the content of Carol's speech consisted of maternal type prohibitions and comments about crying, such as "She likes to cry," "She's cute when she cries." Tina's speech remained infantile and coquettish, but she was at times quite assertive verbally. We were still unable to clearly assess her intellectual capacity; she often had difficulty in comprehension, and in such situations immediately regressed to infantile speech and behavior. Kate was just beginning to speak when her mother removed her from therapy. On the few occasions that we have had a speech therapist for the group, Annaletta, Bob, and Walter have shown the most interest and seemed anxious to please and to learn.

IV · The Mothers' Group:

First Two Years

Mrs. T.—Mother of Tina
Mrs. M.—Mother of Mike
Mrs. B.—Mother of Bob
Mrs. W.—Mother of Walter

The mothers' therapy group consisted of the mothers of Tina, Mike, Bob, and Walter, who met once a week for 90 minutes with one of the authors (RWS). Annaletta's mother was seen individually for eight months and later joined the second mothers' group. During the first half of the Tuesday children's group therapy, the mothers sat around, played bridge, went shopping, or ignored each other. Then they met in the waiting room and all went down together with the therapist to a small, windowless observation room, eight feet square, with a mirror ("one-way screen" with an observer behind it) opposite the door. The room was furnished with a wooden table about the size of a card table, upon which a microphone was placed, and five wooden chairs. There were bright fluorescent lights in the ceiling.

From the first meeting, the four mothers were intensely interested in therapy and made conscientious efforts to understand and alter their interactions with their psychotic children. No sessions were missed without realistic reasons, and in spite of the constant frustration and slow progress, they were enthusiastic in their quest for understanding. In the first session the therapist made a statement to the mothers approximately as follows: "I do not know what has caused your child to be ill, and I am not sure that we will ever know. I believe that there is an interaction between you and your child, an interaction which began in the child's infancy, which is continuing in the present and preventing your child from maturing properly, and at the same time causing you untold distress. I believe by our meeting together weekly and talking over events that occur between you and the child, and especially the feelings that accompany such events, we can understand this interaction and help you to alter it, to the advantage of both." Then followed a few questions and answers, then silence.

After several minutes, each mother in turn expressed feelings of guilt and shame over the harm she felt she had done her child, and her doubts that it could be undone. The therapist repeated his statement that he did not know what had caused the illness and was not seeking to establish blame; we were to concern ourselves with what was going on right now (understood in terms of the past), to see if some things might need to be handled differently.

The mothers then related instances of conflict between themselves and their children. The mother's view of the situation was that the child was intentionally bedeviling her and that she was powerless to stop him. Each mother said that she could see no reason for the child's behavior, and that if she *could* understand why he acted this way, then she would be able to make him stop.

The next few sessions followed a similar pattern: Expressions of guilt were followed by descriptions of interactions in which the child "purposely tormented" the mother. The group resistance was thus initially manifested by an implied definition of *their* goal in therapy, as if to say, "We are here to understand our children. Once we understand what their behavior means, we can control it and deal with it." The remainder of their fantasy was that the mother was to report what her child did, the therapist in turn would explain what the behavior meant, and the mother could then go home and make the child behave properly. Instead, the therapist's response was to ask each mother how she thought her child *felt*, how she herself felt, and what she ordinarily did to cope with the situation. These questions produced anxiety and frustration and led to affective recall of other events in the mother-infant relationship. We were then able to get a much more detailed and meaningful history of this early rlelationship and to see its continuation into the current mother-child interaction. One mother's recall of an event, affectively recited in the permissive atmosphere of the group, seemed to stimulate recall in another, then another.

Ambivalence and identification were prominent in these mothers' attitudes toward their children. Their intensely hostile feelings were verbalized in such words as, "I could have murdered him." "I felt like bashing his head against the wall." "I was so mad I couldn't speak." These statements appeared both in the mothers' recital of present-day events and in their recall of events of the past. There were also many instances in which the mother handled the child as she had wished to be treated by her own mother. Both in present and past situations the mothers displayed a remarkable lack of awareness of the child's actual needs, responding instead to their own needs, which they mistook for the child's. During the child's early infancy the mother could vicariously gratify her own needs in this way, but once the child became physically

able to separate himself from the mother, her need for symbiosis was compromised, and a struggle between mother and
child developed. The mother designated the child as "sick,"
and sought medical advice as to how to restore "health."
When other measures failed, psychiatric help was sought as a
last resort; but here too, the mothers did not get the kind of
"help" they anticipated, and angry frustration resulted. The
intensity of these mothers' anger was remarkable, and it remained the main focus of therapy for the first eighteen months
of group meetings.

The group's initial view of the purpose of therapy was dealt
with as a resistance, and soon true group formation occurred,
with the expected transference manifestations. The therapist
was now seen as an ungiving mother, and the focus of the
conflict shifted from mother *vs.* child to mother *vs.* therapist.
Mrs. M. presented herself as a highly competent, mature individual with utter disdain for the childishness of others, who
therefore deserved the therapist's love and attention. Mrs. W.
pictured herself as a deprived child who had suffered under
an incompetent mother and a ridiculous father, and was now
married to an inadequate husband; having lacked so much, she
felt she now deserved gratification of her childhood fantasy of
being a little princess. Mrs. T. portrayed herself as a little
child who had been bad and deserved punishment, but since
she had already punished herself, felt she should be rewarded
with love and affection. Mrs. B. presented herself as an ideal
example of virtuous self-denial, in that she had never had an
angry thought toward anyone; her only wish was to have nosey
psychiatrists get out of her life so that she could enjoy the
rewards she deserved and had so long striven for.

There was never enough time in a session for all the mothers
to have their say, and sibling rivalry began to appear. When an
interpretation was made to the group, each mother reacted as
if it applied to the others, but not to herself, and took this
as a sign of special approval by the therapist. Similarly, when

an interpretation could not be rejected, the mother reacted as if it were a sign of disapproval and then made renewed efforts to please the therapist. As therapy proceeded, and the initially anticipated gratification from the therapist failed to materialize, anger and frustration mounted. During this period the group reacted as though the way to gain their ends was to annihilate the opposition, the "siblings" in the group, and they began vehement attacks on one another's defenses. The target shifted within each session and from one session to another, but someone was always being "ganged up on" and vigorously attacked. They ultimately verbalized their frustration to the therapist thus: "You may be a good mother to those kids, but you are a damned poor mother to us." Following this, they presented two group dreams involving a death wish toward the "therapist-mother": Mrs. W.: "You had taken me to a circus and when we got there you were sick and I thought you were going to die;" Mrs. B.: "I dreamed you died too." Each mother laughingly made comments about the therapist's failure to meet their needs.

The mothers then tried to reach out to their husbands to gain some gratification, but this was met by increased aloofness and distancing maneuvers. But the husbands could not keep themselves completely away from these determined women, and soon both mothers *and* fathers were seeking the formation of a fathers' group. (When this group did form the mothers anticipated some change favorable to themselves. But again they were frustrated, for the fathers were not seeking to change, but rather to get help in coping with their wives.)

The subsequent sessions were of two kinds, one in which rage was verbalized affectively but without insight, and a second type in which they avoided attacking each other's defenses. Generally, however, the group rage became more intense, and at its height, Mrs. T. became overtly psychotic (mostly limited to the group meetings) and Mrs. B. teetered on the verge of psychosis. We later learned that Mrs. T.'s husband had undergone a vasectomy while on overseas duty, which together with his absence probably precipitated this severe reaction.

Since the group appeared to be merely abreacting their feelings and were unable to observe and integrate their behavior, it was felt that the intensity of the situation should be reduced. Consequently, coffee and doughnuts were served at the end of the first hour of the 90-minute session. This had the desired effect, but added other complications, which had to be dealt with in later sessions.

The mothers used the "coffee break" primarily as a safety valve. The first hour of each session became a series of tantrums, and the last half hour a social gathering. The therapist accepted the tantrum, but pointed out the sudden change. Then the tantrums disappeared, and a teasing, joking discussion about the therapist himself ensued. This behavior was also pointed out to them, and its meaning questioned. The group finally verbalized various fantasies as follows: "We can't bite the hand that feeds us"; "If we continue to be naughty children, he will stop giving us goodies"; "He feeds us to show us that he still loves us in spite of our naughtiness"; and finally, "He got too frightened of our rage, feared we would all go crazy, and had to do something to stop it." At this point it was possible for the therapist to admit that their anger had been pretty hard to take, and that the offering of food was in an effort to reduce the intensity of feelings and to give them an opportunity to look at their feelings, rather than merely to vent them indiscriminately. Then the group developed the additional function of an "observing ego," and further therapeutic progress took place. They focused now on the anger which they experienced consciously, but as a totally unacceptable part of themselves. They tried to get rid of it by expressing it in safe situations, hiding it temporarily and "dumping" it elsewhere, and of course taking it out on the children, husband, group members, and the therapist. After becoming more fully aware of the extent of this anger and its power to create undesirable situations, they eventually sought to discover more about its origin and nature.

For the next six months, the mothers concerned themselves with realistic observations of their behavior at home and in the group. They attempted to correlate this behavior with childhood experiences and with their fantasied expectations of life.

Then role-playing [11] in the group became prominent and was strenuously used as resistance to further progress. Mrs. W. complained loudly and bitterly that she was unable to cope with problems and sought help for everything that happened in her chaotic life; she acted like a spoiled, demanding child, expressing the aggressive pregenital instinctual demands of the group, a position which was bitterly attacked by the "group superego." Mrs. T. took a sexually provocative role, letting her skirt slide above her knees, and sitting so that her thighs were exposed. Her dress, make-up, coiffure, and gestures were a caricature of a girl flagrantly "on the make." The group, however, quite ignored her behavior for several months. Mrs. B.'s behavior was that of a greedy child who verbalized the group's envy of wealthy or fortunate people, and anyone who they considered had more than they did. Mrs. M. was permitted by the group to represent the leader who knew all the answers to her own problems and those of the others. She became the ego ideal of the group. The "ideal" role, the "sexual" role, and the "envious" role were condoned, rationalized, or ignored, and, while the "spoiled child" role was attacked in the person of Mrs. W., no attempt was made to change her, and no one sought to take this role away from her. All the roles were externalized and compartmentalized within the group and, as such, resisted interpretive influence until the increasing frustration of narcissistic wishes once again reached an intolerable intensity. At that point, Mrs. M.

11. S. H. Foulkes and E. J. Anthony (1957), *Group Psychotherapy: The Psychoanalytic Approach* (Baltimore, Penguin Books).

demonstrated by her behavior that she was less than perfect; Mrs. W. showed herself much less chaotic and demanding than she had been encouraged to appear; and Mrs. B. recognized that her envy of others brought her constant unhappiness and frustration. Mrs. T.'s behavior persisted, and it was only when it was pointed out to the group that no one but Mrs. T. seemed to have any sexual feelings or fantasies that some group blind spots became evident. Thus, the role-playing was finally exposed, and each "player" began to see the other members of the group more realistically.

Near the twentieth month of therapy, an exhibition of finger paintings was held, and paintings of Mrs. M., B., and W. were shown. (Mrs. T. had refused to participate in finger painting.) The paintings of Mrs. M. (the "ideal" one) were praised by outsiders, but her response to this revealed to the others her selfishness and egocentricity. She became less than "ideal" and when their own paintings were displayed for several weeks in the hospital corridor, Mrs. B. and Mrs. W. for the first time saw themselves as her equal.

Mrs. T. resented the interpretation of her sexual provocativeness and angrily accused the group of "using" her. She intimated that they all had secret desires toward the therapist, and said that she was tired of being exploited by people. She related a lifetime of incidents in which she had been ill-used by others and said that this exploitation continued currently in her marriage. She felt she had been done an injustice, and would do no more work in therapy until the wrongs were righted—she referred both to her husband in actuality and the therapist in the transference. Attempts were made to gain her associations as to what would right the wrongs, but she refused to say.

The group spent several sessions verbalizing sexual fantasies. The initial fantasies were of idealized males (representing the therapist), followed by sexual fantasies towards highly depreciated males who they said represented their husbands.

Discussion of the sexual fantasies revealed that they represented dependency conflicts which had become sexualized, a transformation of the "good and bad mother" concept. The idealized male is the "good mother," who gratifies all wishes, while the depreciated male is the "bad mother" who is unable to gratify any wishes adequately.

At this point the behavior of the group could be epitomized as being like that of a small child toward her mother, a child who demands that the mother love her exclusively and fulfill all her wishes. It was possible to point out to each member the ways in which they individually sought to gain this end, and how by role-playing they had sought it collectively as a group. In the discussion that followed, they recognized how they had tried to attain the coveted "mother-child" relationship in their own marital relationships and later by identification with their own children. They became aware of the similarity between their own behavioral patterns and those of the children, and numerous correlations were revealed. Mrs. M. said that Mike is coy and seductive in his demanding behavior, and he pouts, acts indifferent, and refuses to listen when he is frustrated; she recognized the fact that she behaves in much the same way under similar circumstances. Mrs. W. spoke of Walter's disregard of the rights of others, his grabbing whatever he wants, and his tantrums when frustrated; she vividly described how she wished to do the same. Mrs. B. mentioned Bob's clinging behavior, his attitude of innocence, and his sly attacks on others, and correlated this with her own behavior towards relatives, neighbors, and friends. The group pointed out to Mrs. T. the seductively provocative behavior of Tina, and identified it as a replica of her own; once again, however, she insisted that this was the way things were to be, and that she would not alter her behavior until her husband altered his. Again the group demanded that she verbalize what it was her husband was to alter and attempted to point out to her the significance of her seductive behavior. Mrs. T. exchanged angry words with the group and would not listen to their suggestions and interpretations. The group attacked her for this and suggested that she leave. She insisted that she no longer needed therapy, which she said was boring and repetitious. This was interpreted to her as being her characteristic self-destructive, defiant behavior. She remained in the group, but acted as if she stayed only to prove herself right. Thus her role changed from that of a sexually provocative child to one of defiance, in which she was determined to get her own way even at the risk of destroying herself. At the time, we did not fully recognize that this behavior was another manifestation of role-playing: Mrs. T. was acting out the group's unconscious resistance to change.

V · Correlations between Mothers'

and Children's Groups

An intriguing aspect of this project was the correlation of the behavior in the children's group with the unconscious group fantasy of the mothers. Similarly, the behavior of the individual child became understandable in terms of the unconscious wishes of his mother. Here the true implications of the word "symbiosis" became apparent. Although we had expected that something of this sort would occur, we were repeatedly surprised to find the evidence so convincing.

The dynamics of Mrs. T.'s behavior can be summarized as follows: "Badness" (sexualized aggression) leads to guilt, followed by self-punishment and submission to the mother's will, followed by dependent gratification. Such a pattern was readily available to her through identification with her own mother. She connected her original "badness" with her father's imprisonment, which she believed resulted from her wishes toward him, both sexual wishes and hostility because of his interference with her relationship with her mother. The theme of her subsequent life as a child with her mother and grandmother became that of atonement for her fantasied misdeed. She later repeated the same pattern in the sequence of rape, forgiveness, and acceptance by husband, and masochistic sub- mission to her husband. The birth of each child caused a similar repetition of the pattern, and Tina was a constant re- minder to Mrs. T. of her "badness" and need for punishment. The cycle reached a climax when her husband had a vasectomy overseas; she became psychotic, having delusions that he had been killed and that she was responsible for his death. She repeated the cycle in fantasy just before his return: she went to a party, became intoxicated, and was taken home by a college boy. She awoke the next morning with amnesia for everything that had happened after she left the party. She had the fantasy that she had been raped and was pregnant, and imagined how her husband would react when she told him.

Mrs. T.'s behavior in the group therapy illustrates further repetitions of this pattern: she presented herself as a "bad little girl" who must atone for her badness by subjugating herself to the will of others. Her mannerisms were sexually aggres- sive. She dressed provocatively and always sat opposite the therapist, repeatedly exposing herself by lifting her skirt and crossing her legs. She strutted about in a teasing, flirtatious manner and had a way of batting her eyes reminiscent of the "flapper" of the 1920's. In the group she described how she repeatedly found herself in potentially sexualized situations with men and wondered how men could so misinterpret her actions. Her unconscious drive to bring about rejection as a form of punishment (with the eventual goal of achieving love and forgiveness by confession to a parental figure) did not alter during her therapy. This reached a climax when the group demanded she leave the group, the last in a long line of recapitulations of the early "rejection" by her mother and father: her aunt, grandmother, and later the boy who raped her, and now periodically her husband, all have rejected her.

Tina imitated her mother's mannerisms to a comical

degree, such as strutting, pursing her mouth, and batting her eyelids with up-turned eyes. Her teasing, flirtatious manner while doing such things as mouthing objects, masturbating, and exploring the boys' penises suggests that she was trying to gain control of the situation by compelling attention, and there was clearly an aura of coy naughtiness in her manner. She also often lay in the middle of the floor in a way which invited the aggression of the other children, and she managed to get stepped on, shoved, and fallen over repeatedly. With each such "insult" she would lift her tear-filled eyes to the therapist and stretch out her arms, communicating her wish to be picked up and cuddled. When instead she received an explanation of her behavior, she had a tantrum. This seemed strikingly similar to some of her mother's behavioral sequences, including naughtiness, pitifulness, and frustrated rage.

Mrs. M. presented herself as "intellectual," sophisticated, highly competent, and disdainful of the childishness of others. Intellectually, she admitted some trivial faults in herself, her husband, and her marriage, but when more basic and realistic deficiencies were pointed out to her by other group members, she reacted defensively and with anger. It was soon learned that the birth of her younger sister had disrupted her idyllic union with her mother, and that she had suffered intense feelings of inadequacy and inferiority. To make up for being displaced, she boosted her own self-esteem by ridiculing the "childishness" of her sister, and in this way she was able to pretend that everything was just as it used to be, everything was perfect. She readily intellectualized paradoxes and denied the reality that she was actually no longer the only child. In later life she developed unrealistic needs to be the perfect wife and mother, married to a perfect husband, and presenting to the world a perfect family; any imperfections were rejected or denied. She abhorred any show of childishness or child-like dependency, either in herself or members of her family. Anger and hate, potentially disruptive of idyllic harmony, were similarly rejected. Although she admitted lack of sexual satisfaction, she insisted that her marriage was so ideal for her that this aspect of her life was of negligible importance. In group sessions she stated, "I have often thought of having sexual relations with men who I thought could satisfy me, but in order to do this I would have to *own* them." The marriage seemed like that of two people who play at being grown-ups, but are unable to communicate real feeling to one another, for fear that real deficiencies might show up which would mar their idyllic existence. Mrs. M. was oblivious of her intense anger, great sexual interest, sexually provocative exhibitionistic behavior, and profound dependency demands. In contrast to Mrs. T., Mrs. M. was sophisticated, subtle, and overtly co-operative. In her verbalizations the unconscious penis interest and the equation breast = penis were evident.

Mike, however, acted out all these feelings for her. His attitude was arrogant, haughty, and completely disdainful of the others in the group. He demanded complete, undivided attention, and praise for his knowledge of squares, triangles, trapezoids, and parallelograms, and his ability to draw beachballs. However, he was exhibitionistic to a comic degree, in that he grimaced, postured, jumped about, and shouted expletives like, "My daddy has a big penis." Like his mother, he seemed unaware of angry feelings, and like her, he seemed to equate overt anger with loss of control.

Mrs. W. verbalized her "little princess" fantasy quite early in therapy. Historically, she had once occupied such a position in relation to her mother, but was displaced by the illness of her older sister and the birth of her younger sister. Mrs. W. tried to transfer this relationship to her father, but without success. Her subsequent behavior had as its goal the reconstitution of the early mother-child relationship, but the inevitable frustration led to intense rage. Through identification with Walter she could obtain vicarious gratification, but only so long as no actual demands were made on her in return. Once

Walter was able to separate from her physically, she felt as though she had once again been barred from the dependent gratification which she "deserved." In the group she related fantasies of displacing Grace Kelly, Queen Elizabeth, and Mrs. Kennedy. She ruthlessly "annihilated" her real and fantasied opponents, histrionically, with laughing and apologies, but with impressive intensity. She paraded the inadequacies of her husband and parents before the group, devalued and "destroyed" them, and replaced them with such grand people as Prince Rainier, Prince Philip, and President Kennedy. She complained that she did not get enough in the group, and asked for more time, more activities, financial help, and finally an individual therapist. When attacked by other members of the group for her selfish demands, she withdrew into surly silence as if she had been unjustly criticized. However, she usually returned quickly to the fray with renewed vigor in her demands.

Walter's behavior was like that of a "little prince" whose every demand must be fulfilled without effort of his own, and whose every impulse may be acted on without self-restraint. He was very greedy about objects and food; when he wanted another child's toy of the moment, he simply took it with an arrogant air which soon earned him the nickname "King Walter." His laughing attacks on the other children and the therapist were reminiscent of his mother's attacks on the members of her therapeutic group. Similarly, when his actions met with restraint or counterattack, he acted crushed, withdrew to a corner, and sucked his thumb for a while, but soon returned with new vigor to pursue his usual aims.

Mrs. B. portrayed herself as an innocent victim of unjust circumstances due primarily to the machinations of others. She insisted on recognition of her true worth as a devout Christian and expected to achieve the good life which she felt she deserved. She disavowed all such characteristics as hate, envy, jealousy, laziness, and gossip, and she repeatedly stated that she had no such attributes, since she had been brought up in a good Christian home. It became apparent that the birth of her younger brother when she was two years old had been a profound narcissistic wound, and that she had subsequently given up all such impulses as undesirable and had become a "good little girl" in the hope of regaining the lost mother-infant relationship. She seemed to have fulfilled this goal in her marriage to a successful businessman from the "right side of the tracks," but the illusion was soon shattered by his multiple depressive episodes and eventual hospitalization; this not only blighted her dependency on him, but forced *her* to act like a mother toward *him*. It seems likely that she blamed Bob for her loss of dependent gratification, in that Mr. B.'s first depressive episode occurred within six months of Bob's birth. It is also likely that she misidentified Bob with her younger brother, so that repressed rage was reactivated and directed toward Bob. But Mrs. B. herself did not feel angry, envious, or jealous; these "bad" emotions were attributed to Bob. She frequently talked about shopping trips and visits to in-laws and neighbors in which she vividly detailed the destructive things she "knew" that Bob would do during such outings. When her certainty about these events was questioned, she defensively attacked the interrogator, demanding to be permitted to live her life without psychiatrists prying into it. She blandly denied anger or envy, and hinted that others were angry and jealous of her, reactions which are reminiscent of a paranoid personality.

Bob related to the other children with sly but violent attacks, then looked as though he vaguely expected retaliation, but seemed incredulous when it actually occurred. He entered the room at each session with a sly grin on his face, then viciously attacked any child who seemed to have or to be getting something he didn't have. He would then retreat to a corner uneasily, but when one of the group attacked him in retaliation for his original aggression, he would say, "Why Mike hit Bob"?

Although Annaletta's mother was not a member of the mothers' group, she often stopped the therapist in the hallway to talk about herself. Her remarks were blandly irrelevant, in contrast to the anger evident in her facial expressions. This was not identical to, but highly reminiscent of, Annaletta's gibberish. Mrs. A's way of "trapping" people was also very similar to Annaletta's technique of "fascination," holding one's attention firmly, yet keeping one at a distance. Annaletta's hoarding behavior with small toys and her peculiar way of giving them up has been interpreted as a struggle between physical starvation and loss of love. If she relinquishes the objects she feels she will starve physically, but if she continues to hoard, she will be starved for love. Her mother's ambivalent behavior toward the Welfare Department and her therapist was strikingly similar.

It was repeatedly demonstrated that the children's behavior altered only after the unconscious fantasy in the mothers' group was verbalized and interpreted. Here are a few outstanding instances: The children's group was much more aggressively hostile on Friday than on Tuesday (the day the mothers' group met). On Fridays, the mothers brought the children earlier and were late in picking them up after the session. They were confronted with these facts, and the ensuing discussion led to their verbalizing their anger at the therapist for giving more time to the children than to them. They admitted that the early arrival and late pick-up of the children was to punish the therapist and make him suffer. Once this material was verbalized and correlated with childhood memories of feeling that their parents favored others, the children's behavior altered to the point that Friday hardly differed from Tuesday. Whenever an impending holiday, vacation, or absence for professional reasons was announced, the mothers reacted overtly with stoical "understanding," but the children almost immediately began hostile, aggressive action toward the therapists. Only when the mothers verbalized their angry feelings about the therapist's leaving, did the children's behavior change. As another example, the mothers were informed at the start of treatment that observers would occasionally be present behind the "one-way screen," and they made very little comment at the time. However, the children's behavior in front of the mirror became increasingly exhibitionistic. They often turned out the lights in the room, which enabled them to see into the observing room, which was imperfectly darkened. We answered their questions about this truthfully. After about six months of therapy, however, the exhibitionistic behavior was remarkable and prompted the comment, "They are acting like monkeys in a cage, performing for visitors." At the same time, it was noted that in their own interview room, the mothers were trying to sit with their backs to the mirror and were turning their chairs sideways to accomplish this. Then two events brought the whole problem into focus: A medical school class was being held in the observation room next to the children's group room, and the students were leaving at the same time that the mothers were bringing the children for their session; the mothers observed talk (and no doubt laughter) during this exodus. On another occasion, as they came to pick up the children after a session, the door to the observing room was open, and they saw several doctors observing the children through the screen. In the following two sessions the mothers were particularly hostile toward the therapist, psychiatry and psychiatrists, the medical school and doctors in general. The therapist commented that the position of their chairs and their attacking him must be somehow related to the fact that there was an observer behind the mirror. They then verbalized their fantasies of being watched. The outstanding fantasy was of monkeys in a zoo. They felt that both they and their children were being laughed at, criticized, and used for the entertainment of the doctors and others. They accused the therapist of not telling them about observers, but at the same time denied curiosity about the people who might be watching. They only partially verbalized their own exhibitionistic wishes, but after this session, the exhibitionistic behavior of the children's group diminished markedly. Of course sporadic individual exhibitionistic behavior continued, just as in the case of the mothers.

Another interesting kind of correlation was noted: Often it seemed that when a child was being treated in a certain way by the children's group, the child's mother was being similarly treated by the mothers' group. When Mrs. W. was being attacked in the mothers' group, Walter was usually being attacked in the children's group. Similarly, the behavior and attitudes of the children's group towards Tina and Bob could be correlated with the attitudes and behavior of the mothers' group toward Mrs. T. and Mrs. B. during the period when they were, respectively, psychotic and nearly psychotic. This was manifested by attitudes of extreme caution and protectiveness toward both mothers and similarly toward the two children.

These correlations strengthened our view that the child often acted out the mother's unconscious fantasies, and this increased our understanding of the mother's need for a symbiotic relationship with the child. Only by assisting the mother to verbalize her feelings and recognize them as her own could the child's behavior be altered. Accordingly we repeatedly formulated the dynamic interaction between mother and child as one in which the child acts out the unacceptable unconscious impulses of the mother; and that through such action the mother gains vicarious gratification of her wishes, and through the external struggle with the child externalizes her internal conflict.

Looked at from this point of view, it is evident that the child is in an impossible bind. By non-verbal means the mother communicates unmistakable commands to act out these impulses, but at the same time she verbally forbids them and punishes the child for his compliance. She expects him to be a dependent infant, yet she verbally demands that he be mature. The goal of therapy in the mothers' group is to assist her to recognize her unconscious wishes, to accept them as her own, and to deal with them herself, rather than trying to gain fulfillment of them through the child. Once this has taken place, the child is no longer required to deal with his mother's paradoxical impulses, and can begin learning how to deal with his own. We felt that this problem was epitomized by some of the children's remarks: "Dr. Speers, why the ghost after Bob? What Bob done that ghost after him? Is Bob a bad boy that ghost mad at him?"; "Dr. Speers, say Bob not bad for taking off clothes. Why Bob get spanked for taking off clothes if Bob not bad?"; "Why Bob take off clothes?"; "Why Bob hit Tina?"; Mike says, "Babies can't talk, babies can't play, babies can't eat. Mike wants to be a big boy, not a baby." "Dr. Speers, Mike doesn't want to get mad. Mike wants to be happy, don't want to get mad." "I want to play with big toys, not baby toys." All these statements had a quizzical tone, as if the source of the impulse to be bad or to be a baby were felt to come from the external world. We had the impression that the children felt obliged to behave in a manner inimical to at least some of their own desires.

VI · The Fathers' Group:

First Two Years

Group therapy with the fathers of the psychotic children was a difficult project, in that each man had long used isolation techniques which effectively prevented significant emotional relationships, let alone group formation. Themselves the children of immature, narcissistic mothers, these men had all suffered serious dependency frustration since early childhood. Fearing that their powerful ambivalence would destroy the anaclitic object, they had withdrawn enough to avoid alienating their mothers, but at the cost of alienating themselves. They reduced their conscious oral demands to a minimum, and were in consequence seriously "underfed" emotionally. As children, they had withdrawn from their mothers, and as adults they kept physically and emotionally isolated from their wives and children. Similarly, group sessions were marked by physical absences, emotional isolation when physically present, obsessive rumination, and compulsive behavior.

The fathers were not aware of these personality problems, however, and did not seek therapy for themselves, but were really pushed into it by their wives. Let us review the dynamics of the mothers' group, which had been operating for nine months before the fathers' group was formed: Early in their group therapy, the mothers sought to gratify, through the therapist, their unconscious and narcissistic dependency needs. When he refused to be an all-giving mother, they sought gratification from their husbands, then bitterly complained about how inadequate their husbands were, and finally put pressure on them to enter therapy and (presumably) change in the direction of greater adequacy. They acquiesced, mostly to placate their wives, and not because of any insight into their deficiencies as husbands and fathers. But their old patterns of emotional isolation, which had enabled them to remain aloof from their mothers, wives, and children, now continued in the group therapy. They formed a loose, affable, guarded association with one another, like strangers on a train, and seemed to get from this some minimal dependency gratification and mutual support, as long as feelings remained tepid. But when strong or "dangerous" feelings, especially negative ones, appeared, they retreated sharply, even to the extent of prolonged absence from the sessions, always rationalized as due to unavoidable business obligations.

Mr. W. talked obsessively about intellectualized material, but whenever feelings appeared, in himself or others, he would fall asleep. Similarly, Mr. B. could gain and hold control of the group by long rambling discussions of his work and his relations with the office personnel, but when emotionally charged topics were introduced, he would become silent and withdrawn. Mr. M. attended sessions infrequently and tried to monopolize the group with stories of how important he was; he would then dart away from the group and remain absent for three or four weeks. Mr. T's tactic was to appear about every five weeks, drop a verbal "bomb," (consisting of violent criticism of his wife or other members of the group, couched in outhouse phrases), leave the session, and then return weeks later to repeat the performance. Mr. B. manipulated everyone by his constant threats to become depressed (recalling previous hospitalizations) and used this to monopolize the group session or to get time alone with the therapist. Mr. W. rarely missed a session, and both he and his wife spent much time criticizing those who failed to attend regularly or were not properly grateful to the doctors and other participants in the program. He constantly appealed for help with his family problems, but demonstrated his unconsciously negativistic attitude toward the whole proceedings by talking about his bowels, smelling his watch, and falling asleep.

With personnel turnover, the fathers' group during the first two years had altogether three therapists, all of whom felt intensely frustrated in trying to deal with the fathers' absenteeism and general resistance, which kept the therapist (as perhaps the wife and child) constantly frustrated, but always enticed with the possibility of eventual participation. All the therapists thought the fathers were capable people who could utilize therapy, with regular attendance and active participation, but the constant struggle to get them to attend impeded the group in getting on with the therapy. After 20 months of therapy, patient and persistent interpretations plus gradually increased family interactions resulted in the fathers' recognizing that the isolation technique is a defense, and they subsequently became more willing to relinquish it and to enter more actively into therapy.

Study of the fathers gave very little concrete data about the families' problems. It was our impression, however, that the emotional isolation was at the forefront of the problem, and that when its defensive nature was completely analyzed, group formation would take place in therapy. Most importantly, group interaction within the family would occur, the problem of the psychologically absent father would be resolved, and many of the basic emotional needs of both parents and child would be met. The reduction of the mothers' unrealistic de-

mands on the fathers was, we felt, already of great importance in permitting the fathers to begin to participate in rewarding group interactions. The fathers had less need to
isolate themselves, as the children became more human and
accessible, giving these men more self-esteem in their role as
fathers, which allowed them to face more courageously the
possible criticism of the therapist and other members of the
group. This in turn allowed them to use less denial of their
own problems and to face some of their deficiencies.

We were unable to get much tangible evidence about feelings
on this score from the fathers, but we inferred that their
tendency to a rather wistful aloofness, withdrawal and isolation
stemmed from their childhood relationship with their mothers,
who had dominated and coerced them. Probably following the
pattern of their own passive and depreciated fathers, they
preserved their identity by emotional withdrawal from the
mother, and perhaps by angry pouting. They reacted similarly
to any angry reproach from their wives. There developed patterns of neurotic interaction in the marriage characterized by
aloofness, sulking, or absence on the part of the husbands,
and conscious suppression (and sometimes unrestricted expression) of anger by the wives. Several of the couples could
maintain a semblance of normal emotional interaction as long
as no frightening negative feelings arose, but when the wife's
angry demands were manifested, the husband, to avoid being
openly "disobedient," reacted by evasive tactics reminiscent of
a covertly reluctant little boy. We surmise that this reaction
had also been used against the mother in childhood and that its
use against the group therapist's "demand" that feelings be
faced, indicated a predominantly maternal transference in
therapy.

VII · Propositions

Our theoretical frame of reference regarding childhood psychosis may be summarized as follows: The psychotic child and his parents are psychologically committed to maintain a symbiotic relationship between mother and child which precludes regression of the child to an earlier phase of development, the phase of autism (in which there is no personal identity, no distinction between self and non-self, and no experience of the mother as something apart from self) but also precludes advancement of the child to a more mature phase of development, the phase of separation-individuation, (in which there is real awareness of complete physical and psychological separateness of mother from child, with realization of separate identities, ego boundaries, impulse and affect control, and complete and distinct body image). The fixity of the symbiotic relationship is related to its source, an equilibrium between strongly opposed tendencies towards fusion and separation, both of which generate intense anxiety if permitted to dominate the relationship. A compromise is made, in which some degree of personal identity experience is preserved, but ego boundaries are shared, along with control of impulse and affect. The child magically controls the distance that he perceives to exist between himself and mother.

Although the situation is in reality most unsatisfactory, it does serve a defensive function and hence is necessary to both mother and child; it is also essential to father and perhaps gratifying to some other family members. The total situation is psychotic in that the reality of physical and psychological separateness is denied. Resistance to alteration of the status quo is monumental, stemming not only from the child, but from the mother and father as well. These psychotic interactions begin early in the child's life and persist regardless of physical maturation and environmental change.

In order to communicate the essence of our therapeutic method, we will divide our discussion into three aspects of our experience in this program. In this chapter we will review and discuss the opening phase of therapy with the children. In Chapter VIII we will discuss the "three-ring circus" of childhood symbiotic psychosis from the standpoint of the child's ego structure, the mother's personality, and the neurotic interaction of the family. Finally, in Chapter IX we will summarize the progress of group therapy during the third and fourth years and discuss these later phases of therapy in terms of the growth of the child's ego, dissolution of the mother-child symbiosis, and changes in the family dynamics.

It is our thesis, in agreement with Mahler and Furer [12] that therapy with the psychotic child can be initiated only in the framework of a relationship which reconstitutes a benign, gratifying early mother-child symbiosis. It is our contention, however, that the concept of "therapeutic symbiosis" is not restricted to a one-to-one relationship between a mothering figure and a psychotic child, but that in a group situation, a

12. M. S. Mahler and M. Furer (1960), Observations on research regarding the "symbiotic syndrome" of infantile psychosis, *Psychoanalytic Quarterly*, 29:317–327.

"group ego" can serve as one-half of a symbiotic relationship, with the individual child as the junior partner. Similarly, we feel that separation-individuation from the group ego occurs in the same manner as from the therapist-"mother" in the traditional one-to-one therapeutic relationship. The initial problem in either form of therapy is to penetrate the autistic defenses and establish a non-pathological symbiotic relationship. The next phase consists of fostering a gradual separation-individuation process in this new, benign symbiotic relationship. In traditional one-to-one therapy, the usually lengthy initial phase consists of gradual penetration of the autistic barrier and the development of a trusting symbiosis wherein the strong, intact ego of the therapist is "borrowed" by the child. Because the therapist has no wish to perpetuate the symbiosis for personal need satisfactions, it is possible for separation-individuation to take place in due time. In the group therapy technique, penetration of autistic defenses is relatively rapid and is quickly followed by group formation, which in our view, leads to the development of a "group ego" (comprised of all the children, the therapists, and the physical environment) which then serves as the "other half" of each child's symbiotic relationship.

It is important for the reader to understand that we are using the term "autistic defense" to denote a variety of behaviorisms including mute withdrawal; empty, affectless clinging to adults; repetitive twirling of self or toy; bizarre postures and mannerisms reminiscent of catatonia; and some of the seemingly nonsensical speech patterns. These behaviorisms have seemed to us defensive in nature, serving to bring the symbiotic object (mother) totally under the child's magical control, which prevents the loss of the mother by separation or loss of the self through fusion with the mother. The autistic defense enables the child to control the distance between himself and symbiotic object, even in the physical absence of the mother; it is a mechanism for denying the actual degree of both psychological closeness and physical separateness of mother and child.

When placed in the therapy situation, the children initially responded with enhanced autism. This mutual avoidance was not unexpected, and we assumed that the small size of the room and the children's restless milling around would eventually lead to enough body contact to force them to become aware of the environment and each other. However, there was even more physical contact than expected, and we came to recognize it as purposeful, perhaps an indication of residual interest in object relationships. In addition, the therapists' activities were directed toward interfering with the autistic defensive behavior and trying to thrust reality, not too rudely, on the children. We also felt that the mirror on the wall and the constant playing of music assisted in breaking through the defense. The children repeatedly experienced penetration of this defense by the environmental reality; this was followed by physical protection against the overwhelming panic which usually resulted; this in turn led to a regressed relationship which was permitted and made comfortable. Thus the therapeutic situation provided a safe environment in which the need for the autistic defense was lessened, and a regressed state of symbiosis between the individual child and the total therapeutic environment was instead established. Two additional interventions also aided in decreasing the children's need for autistic defenses: the group therapy of the mothers permitted displacement of the mother *vs.* child conflict to mother *vs.* therapist; and the "mammy" similarly gave both the mother and child some relief from the intensity of their habitual interaction and afforded to the child the possibility of an alternative regressed and non-pathological symbiotic relationship outside the therapeutic group.

Once this safe situation was established and the children were in a regressed, symbiotic relationship, it was important that there should be no significant alteration in the total group;

i.e., the room itself, the structures within, the children and the therapists. Any change in the structure resulted in the resumption of autistic defenses and necessitated the children's re-experiencing the sequence described. We would recommend to others that in the early phases of therapy the entire routine should remain as stereotyped as possible.

The physical restraint techniques which were applied to control the panic (and also subsequent unduly aggressive behavior) were not passively accepted by the children; they resisted actively with crying, kicking, head-banging, and lashing out at the controlling therapist. It was our conviction that the child needed this restraint and that only through real physical contact with a therapist's body could the child give up his infantile omnipotence and accept regression to a "safe" symbiotic relationship. The therapists were constantly alert to the patterns and forces which triggered panic in each child, and could quickly, calmly, and firmly control the child in both self-destructive and unduly aggressive behavior. While the child was being held, the therapist verbalized the reason for the restraint and the desirability of the child's behavior being controlled. As therapy progressed, it became our conviction that this physical control was a desirable interaction, as various children, either behaviorally or verbally, requested such control when their own ability to maintain control was threatened. We believe that the firm and consistent application of these physical controls (which provided tactile, visual and auditory contact) enabled the children to relinquish their fantasies of omnipotence, with a concomitant reduction in their fantasies of annihilation and their projected fantasies of being annihilated themselves.

Mike, Bob, and Walter, the children who exhibited defensive autism, went through the following sequence over the first few months of therapy: autism, penetration of the autism, severe panic, a self-destructive type of tantrum behavior, aggression directed outward but without perceptible goal, and finally goal-directed aggresivity. In each of these phases, physical control—often before the mirror, so as to provide visual perceptions of the situation—and the therapists' verbal statements about the reason for the behavior (and the assurances that it *could* be controlled) resulted in the children's developing internal control over much of their aggresive drives. Annaletta required relatively little physical restraint and seemed able to utilize verbal-visual cues in controlling her intense anxiety and aggression. We felt that Tina's libido and aggressivity were fixated in the feeding situation: the nursing bottle seemed to represent the mother's aggression which Tina was attempting to control omnipotently. When she was offered a bottle which she could ward off and an anxiety-free experience was provided, she began to imitate the other children and was able to participate in the symbiotic relationship with the group.

We provided a female and male therapist in each group therapy session in a conscious effort to imitate the normal family structure. In this framework, we gratified many of the real needs of the children and frustrated most of their psychotic demands. Whenever we were convinced that a child was experiencing a particular affect, we told the child what the feeling was called. We early learned that in their own families, feelings of hate, envy, jealously, destructive impulses, dependency longings, helplessness, and crying were all condemned or denied. We felt the children had considerable confusion about these feelings and that it was important to establish them as known, named, understandable, and acceptable. The therapists were also encouraged to talk about and name some of their own feelings, in order to let the children know what affects normal people have, and to learn that such feelings destroy neither therapist nor child.

It was often noted that any intervention (permission, or verbal or physical prohibition), whether directed toward an individual child or to the group as a whole, resulted in a group reaction in which each child seemed to utilize the experience to some extent. Once the initial anxieties had been effectively dealt with, the children became able to act out their conflicts in play and to verbalize their fantasies, and were amenable to some social pressures. At the same time, it became possible to revise distortions in their fantasies.

The reader will recall that the mothers of Walter, Tina, Bob, and Mike were seen 1½ hours weekly in analytically oriented group therapy over a three-year period. Annaletta's mother is an ambulatory schizophrenic who had irregular individual psychotherapeutic interviews. The fathers of the first four children had weekly 1½-hour group therapy sessions, with irregular attendance for two years. Concurrent observation of child and both parents in these therapeutic groups have led to some understanding of the psychotic child's ego, the mother-child symbiosis, and certain family interactions. To the extent that they may be etiologic for psychosis in the past and for its current perpetuation, and insofar as they may be altered, these factors are worthy of attention.

From the mothers' group, verbalized fantasies and memories, transference phenomena, and psychological events in the group (such as Mrs. T's psychotic episode and the near psychosis of Bob's mother) forced upon us the recognition that in spite of the seemingly adequate adaptations that these women had made in life, all had serious personality defects. In each there was a history of intense family conflicts during childhood, poor peer-group relationships, prolonged periods of emotional isolation, intense feelings of low self-esteem, the use of pathological compensatory mechanisms, and a constant struggle to achieve social adjustment. A group statement by the mothers at the height of a transference frustration summarized the difficulties these women have experienced in life: "The beginning of therapy, the birth of the (now psychotic) child, and the marriage itself are similar in that each seemed to promise relief from a lifetime of immense personal dissatisfaction. In each instance we have been disappointed, and our needs have remained unfulfilled." The group transference was an intensely narcissistic, dependent mother-child situation. The "mother" of this transference pair was divided in two, the therapist being the "good mother" and the husband the "bad mother." The "child" was also split, the "good child" being appropriated by the actual mother, (e.g., Mrs. B.), while the "bad child" role was assigned to the bad, sick, psychotic child (e.g., Bob). When the group therapist attempted to block the projection of "badness" onto the children, the mothers then projected it onto each other, so to speak, and through role-playing in the group effectively prevented the integration of many "bad" impulses into their personalities. We feel that this inability to integrate unacceptable impulses into the mother's personality is of profound importance in the under-standing and therapy of childhood psychosis.

Our information about the fathers is more superficial, but we conclude that as a group they are less disturbed than the mothers. They exhibit moderately severe character disorders which do not permit them to function adequately as husbands and fathers, but enable them to adapt to the prescribed cultural role of a male. Their own fathers are characterized as weak and passive, poor models for masculine identification. Their mothers are pictured as castrating, phallic women who depre-ciate males. These men are experts at defending themselves against threats of castration, by physical and psychic withdrawal from the threatening situation. At the same time, they have excessive dependency wishes which have prevented their emancipation from their mothers in the past and from their wives in the present. In each family the marriage has been fraught with frustration and ambivalence, and yet in only one instance (Tina) was there so much as a mention of divorce. It was into such a family environment that each of our patients were born.

It is not possible to ascertain just how much further "pathology" each child brought into these disturbed marriages. The histories obtained from three mothers, (Mike, Walter, Tina) indicated abnormality in the child from the very beginning of life. The other two mothers (Bob, Annaletta) insisted that the child was "normal" as an infant, but as their therapy progressed, it became evident that all the mothers were erratic historians. What they thought the child needed reflected much more their own fears and fantasies than what a calmer or more objective person might have guessed. For instance, both Mike and Tina were responded to as though crying could indicate only hunger. Mrs. W. reacted to Walter as if he had no needs of his own. Mrs. A. and Mrs. B. were so preoccupied with their own problems that they were quite unable to observe their children's development.

In the present state of our knowledge, it seems fruitless to try to resolve the traditional question of whether psychosis is innate or acquired, which hinges on whether personality defects in the parent *induce* developmental fixations and ego defects, or whether they are the result of maturational lags [13] in the child, to which the parents could not adequately respond. However, our experience with the various groups permits a statement of our theoretical orientation. We recognize the fact that in the genesis of childhood psychosis, certain biological variations are operating, some undeniably normal, such as sex and size, others beyond the elusive boundary of "the range of normal," such as aggressive drive endowment and sensitivity to sound, light, and touch. Similarly, it is possible that there may be innate defects in certain ego functions, notably the functions of integration and reality testing. It seems most logical to assume that we are dealing with two chief variables, the child's innate problems and the mother's personality problems, and that it is the interaction of these

13. L. Bender and A. M. Freedman (1952), A study of the first three years in the maturation of schizophrenic children, *Quarterly Journal of Child Behavior*, 4:245–272.

two variables which leads to the psychotic process in the child. We would add that the mother's problems are materially influenced by her interactions with her husband, other members of her family, and her socio-cultural environment. In any case, the debate over etiology is largely academic, since knowledge of such "causes" of psychosis tells us little about how to treat it. It is well for the therapist to consider all the factors as possible, so that he may keep continuously aware of the multiplicity of variables: the biological defects in the child, the pathology in the mother, the tenacious mother-child symbiosis, the psychologically absent father, and the over-all dynamics of interaction in the family. It is our contention that focusing on these variables can afford the therapeutic leverage necessary to alter the psychosis and the network of pathological reactions and relationships in which it is enmeshed.

VIII · The Three-Ring Circus

THE CHILD: SYMBIOSIS AND PSYCHOTIC EGO

The many authors who have investigated the ego defects of psychotic children have created an attractive array of theoretical formulations, representing different points of approach to the problem.

Hartmann [14] proposes a failure in the ego's capacity for neutralization resulting from a defect in the inherited constitutional apparatus.

Bergman and Escalona [15] mention premature ego formation resulting from a defective stimulus barrier.

Klein [16] hypothesizes a splitting of object and ego which results from introjection of part objects upon which hostile impulses have been projected.

14. H. Hartmann (1953), Contribution to the metapsychology of schizophrenia, *Psychoanalytic Study of the Child*, 8:177–198.

15. P. Bergman and S. K. Escalona (1949), Unusual sensitivities in very young children, *Psychoanalytic Study of the Child*, 3–4:333–352.

16. M. Klein (1946), Notes on some schizoid mechanisms, *International Journal of Psycho-Analysis*, 27:99–110.

Eissler [17] stresses defects in the perceptual system.

Jacobsen [18] speaks of failure of development of ego identification, that is, bodily and mental "self-representations."

Federn [19] mentions the fluctuating ego boundaries.

Des Lauriers [20] emphasizes the defective capacity to experience reality.

We would accept most of these as valid, but wish to present our own assessment (in agreement with Mahler and Gosliner) [21] of the child's ego structure and functioning in terms of his need to participate in the symbiosis. A summary of our reconstructions relating to the ego (in Bob, Mike, Walter, and Annaletta) appears below: this neither includes nor excludes the probability of biological deficit in the child, nor is it specifically concerned with the pathological effects of the mothering one.

The child, for whatever reasons, finds the early mother-infant interaction a traumatic experience. This trauma, although mostly limited to the actual feeding situation, also includes other physical interactions such as cuddling, patting, cooing, and stimulation in general. The trauma occurs in the period of the early mother-child interaction wherein the mother is cathected in part and is understood as something

17. K. R. Eissler (1954), Notes upon defects of ego structure in schizophrenia, *International Journal of Psycho-Analysis*, 35:141–146.

18. E. Jacobsen (1954), Contribution to the metapsychology of psychotic identifications, *Journal of the American Psychoanalytic Association*, 2:239–262.

19. P. Federn (1952), *Ego Psychology and the Psychoses* (New York, Basic Books).

20. A. M. Des Lauriers (1962), *The Experience of Reality in Childhood Schizophrenia*, Monograph Series on Schizophrenia, No. 6, New York, International Universities Press.

21. M. S. Mahler and B. J. Gosliner (1955), On symbiotic child psychosis: genetic, dynamic and restitutive aspects, *Psychoanalytic Study of the Child*, 10:195–212.

outside the self. The child's body image, his ego boundaries, and his sense of identity are in the process of development, but their constancy is contingent on visual, tactile, and auditory contact with the mothering one. Although the experiences of the child are unsatisfying and the concomitant anxiety is great, the symbiotic relationship with mother does permit some uneven ego development to occur. Depending upon the amount of anxiety present in the experiences, some integration of experience is possible: the child may develop precursors of speech, followed by a few words, and may develop certain skills, but whatever development does occur is dependent upon visual, auditory, and tactile contact with the mother. But when the child learns to walk, and by chance moves away from his mother, he suddenly and unprecedentedly finds himself out of such contact with her. Unlike the normal child, who suffers only moderate and decreasing anxiety in this situation, the psychotic child experiences overwhelming panic. The fragile ego, which could exist only in the actual context of the symbiosis, is now threatened with annihilation. The immediate response is to seek out the mother, to re-establish contact. If she is not available, the current level of maturity cannot be maintained, and in the face of intense anxiety, regression is inevitable. This regression is apparent to the mother as anxious clinging, with loss of speech and other skills. Other real separations, as when mother is hospitalized for the birth of a sibling, of course have similar effects.

Repetitions of this experience are frequent, and the attendant anxiety forces the child to develop mechanisms for avoiding the ensuing panic. The primary mechanism is one of regression to that period of life when the child actually had constant, visual, auditory, and tactile contact with the mother —the phase of symbiosis. But once having enjoyed the semblance of ego control, the child can now tolerate symbiosis only if he is completely in charge of it; he uses psychotic defenses to maintain regression and to control its degree. Progression to the previous level of maturity would be experienced as complete separation, with annihilation of self or mother; regression beyond the symbiotic phase to the stage of autism would be experienced as an engulfment by the mother. The child must magically use omnipotent, psychotic maneuvers in order to have complete control over the degree of closeness and separateness from mother.

With Tina's psychosis the situation is different in that the trauma occurred somewhat earlier and was fixating in the sense that it did not permit further development. We would say that the trauma occurred during the normally autistic phase of earliest infancy, prior to the development of sym-biosis. In this instance the libido was limited to the oral zone, and ego awareness was fixated on the feeding experience. The only awareness of self versus not-self occurred when an object was inserted in the child's mouth. But since feeding took place in response to the mother's anxiety and not the child's hunger, the mother was not experienced as a person by the child, but rather as something dangerous and intrusive, to be warded off. However, it was only in this interaction of "something in the mouth," in which the child struggled to control the situation, that there was any degree of differentiating self from not-self. It was as if the child were attempting to actively master a trauma which she had heretofore experienced passively and helplessly—a trauma that had been fixating due to the degree of anxiety and had prevented the establishment of a symbiotic relationship.

The children's behavior (apart from Tina's) at the onset of therapy was understood in terms of the child's need to main-tain a symbiotic relationship that denied the immediate reality situation; a symbiosis that actually existed in the past only; a symbiosis that permitted the child omnipotent control of stimuli, both internal and external, and which was free from the anxiety relating to loss of self or loss of mother, for what-ever reasons. Such a situation could exist only in psychotic fantasy and necessitated massive denial for its maintenance. The children behaved autistically: they were oblivious to the fact of separation from their mothers and to the reality of other children, the adult therapist, and the room and its contents. They failed to respond to external stimuli and their expressionless faces suggested absence of internal affect. At the smallest threat to the maintenance of this situation, the child would initiate activities to restore the status quo. At first such activities were limited to retreat to the farthest corner of the room or turning away from an intrusion. As a threat persisted, the children resorted to other behaviorisms for maintaining the fantasied situation: Walter obtained a stuffed animal and sucked his thumb and twirled his hair; Mike defecated in his pants and rolled on the floor; Bob twirled himself round and round; Annaletta climbed onto the window and mirror sills. We found that each child had his own particular repertory which served to maintain or restore the past symbiosis. These can be classified under several headings: (*1*) autism, with its hallucinatory potential; (*2*) provocative behavior, which at home would compel actual contact with mother: Tina's chewing inedible objects; Bob's turning lights on and off, crying, holding arms outstretched to be picked up, crawling onto laps; Mike's defecating and urinating conspicuously, and doing "forbidden" things; special language usage such as Bob's obsessive questioning, Mike's exhibitionistic utterances and Annaletta's gibberish; (*3*) use of an object in a special manner, (actually a psychotic fetish [22]) a kind of "Instant Mother" which is omnipotently controlled by being put in motion, e.g., wheels, sticks, which are twirled or twiddled, playing in water, sucking thumbs, twirling self around, or manipulating part of the body (hands, lips, mouth) instead of an external physical object; (*4*) use of a motion, action, or activity as though it were a person or thing, such as rocking,

22. M. Sperling (1963), Fetishism in children, *Psychoanalytic Quarterly*, 32:374–392.

bumping, twirling, posturing, and autistic "talking"—these may be merely adjuncts to the imaginary evocation of mother through fantasy or hallucination.

To summarize: we came to understand the phenomenology of childhood psychosis in terms of the child's need to maintain a state of regression in which a *past* symbiosis was recreated. This state is actually a dyssymbiosis [23] in that it is not particularly happy or fruitful, but seems preferable to the anxiety of incipient separation. While escaping the dangers of annihilation through separation, the budding ego is threatened by the alternative danger of engulfment. Autistic, omnipotent behavior maintains the proper degree of regression and controls the extent of closeness to and separation from the mother. In therapy the child made active efforts to induce the adults to behave as his parents did, and if the therapists could not be converted into mother, the child used inanimate objects for the same purpose. It is our belief that the symbiosis, thus recreated, is no more and no less satisfactory in the present than in the past, but that mother and child are fixated at this level of interaction without the possibility of progress.

In therapy, penetration of the autistic defense leads to a new symbiosis of a different kind, a present symbiosis which does not impose the same dangers to the ego through engulfment or annihilation. This is not an abrupt transition, but an often repeated back-and-forth series of experiences, which finally enable the child to accept the *present* "therapeutic symbiosis" and to see it as "safe." Within this newly created symbiosis, the child's ego defects become apparent. We wish to discuss these defects in terms of ego boundaries, impulse and affect control, body image, and personal identity, as they appear in the vicissitudes of the therapeutic symbiosis in group therapy. Examining the psychotic child's ego closely, we found

23. D. W. Abse and J. A. Ewing (1960), Some problems in psychotherapy with schizophrenic patients, *American Journal of Psychotherapy*, 14:505–519.

that it can be scrutinized conveniently from four important standpoints:

1) Ego Boundary—Perception of self and not-self and what differentiates the two. In symbiosis, the ego boundaries include the mother.

2) Body Image—Perception of various body parts as belonging exclusively to the self, and perception of the total body as an integrated whole. In symbiosis, some or all body parts may be regarded by the child as extensions of mother.

3) Impulse and Affect—Perception, control, and coping with internal stimuli, drives, reactions. In symbiosis, these may include intrusive stimuli actually arising from the mother.

4) Identity—Perception of the self as more than body, more than impulse and affect, existing in time as well as space. Associated with recognition of name, and use of "I" and "me" in speech.

We felt that the panic reactions in the early stages of therapy resulted from the loss of all four of these ego components and that much of the ensuing behavior was an attempt to restore them. These ego components are of course indivisibly interrelated, and it is obvious that no bit of behavior relates exclusively to a single one; yet it may be more concerned with one component than another. Some behavior may be ambiguous or confusing to the therapist, seeming at first glance to belong chiefly to one ego function, but actually having a stronger connection with another. For example, we eventually understood the child's biting his hand as an attempt to restore his body image and ego boundaries, and not simply misdirected oral cannibalistic activity. Flailing of the body against the therapist or floor belongs in this same category. In general, we understood all such behavior as part of the child's attempt to restore his omnipotent position of symbiosis. It may seem contradictory to state that such behavior is an attempt to restore both "ego" and "symbiosis." We use the term "dys-symbiosis" to distinguish the psychotic state of affairs from the amiable symbiosis of normal infancy in which the normal ego develops. The dyssymbiosis is by contrast a magical, manipulative interaction between mother and child in which the child magically controls the distance between himself and his mother. It is a kind of symbiosis, yet under the child's control. At the same time it substitutes for, and blocks the development of, the more "progressive" ego components which we have enumerated.

With the establishment of the group symbiosis, the hand-biting, head-banging, and flailing behavior diminished greatly, but ego boundaries were still frequently lost. In the early experiments with the soap-bubble water, a child often became so involved with the material that he seemed to "lose himself" in his activity. This was especially true of Walter, who fre-quently needed the therapist to intervene by physical contact to help him reconstitute his boundaries. Even much later in therapy, when the children used finger paint, they reacted with behavior which we felt indicated a similar loss of ego boundaries and a sort of merging of child, activity, and ma-terial, the child "identifying," so to speak, with the color, the tactile quality, or the physical fluidity of the medium. For instance, Mike would be painting with a neutral color, but gradually his activity would increase in intensity as he added more paint and different colors, until he ended up with a dark, muddy mess. At the same time, he would become ab-sorbed, with a faraway stare, in what seemed like autistic fascination with the activity and his participation in it to a point where we felt sure that he no longer distinguished himself from the messy paint on the paper. Interruption of this activity often evoked extremely aggressive behavior.

In the opening phase of each session, activities were usually unstructured, and we felt that the children's pell-mell, somewhat frantic behavior indicated a threatened loss of ego boundaries. Walter protected himself from this danger, so we thought, by drawing a margin around the edge of his paper, which seemed to symbolize the limits of his ego, and later the group ego. He became anxious if his crayon ever went beyond this margin. We thus recognized the necessity of structuring the play and other routine activities which we felt provided internal support to the individual child and to the group.

By the ninth month of therapy, loss of ego boundaries rarely occurred, even when the interaction among the children was intense. However, boundaries could be loosened and sometimes dissolved by prolonged finger painting activity. We felt that this occurred more readily when the children were under some sort of stress from the home events, or in response to specific colors. In general, once the child could tolerate physical closeness, make visual contact with objects and people, and permit auditory stimuli to enter conscious awareness, ego boundaries became relatively stable and would dissolve only under unusual stress.

Body image manifestations are easier to illustrate, because they provide more objective data than the ego boundary phenomenon just described. Often inanimate objects were used and thus were made to move or rotate (to "make them be alive") but body parts could serve the purpose just as well. We have designated this behavior as psychotic fetishism in which the inanimate object or body part *was* the mother with whom the child could do as he pleased. In his activity with the fetish, he made it move, which served both as proof of "aliveness" and of his omnipotent control. Thus the object satisfied the child's symbiotic requirements. However, once the safe group symbiosis had been established, the children began inspecting their bodies with visible affects of curiosity, interest, and occasional delight. They made trips to the mirror and observed and manually explored the mouth, tongue, teeth, head, and many other parts of the body. The therapist would touch

Fig. 1

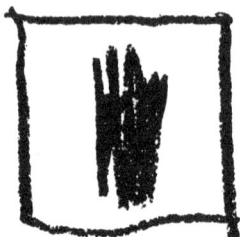

Fig. 2

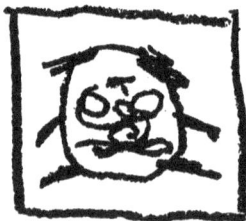

Fig. 3

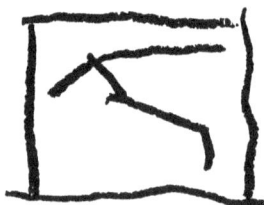

Fig. 4

and name the part which the child was noticing and often his own as well. Thus the child experienced varied but integrated stimuli referring to his body parts: touching and being touched, seeing them directly and in the mirror, hearing them named, and also hearing additional remarks about their location and functions. Visual observation of the co-ordinated action of voice and mouth was a frequent activity before the mirror. The children seemed surprised or fascinated by the discovery that this correlation exists. The development of the body image is most dramatically illustrated in Walter's series of drawings shown above.

Of course, this sort of activity was not wholly without anxiety. Mike was concerned about the possibility of losing teeth or penis, and was ecstatic when he discovered his uvula (always easily visible in the mirror and without infraction of social canons) as if this reassured him of the constancy of pendent parts. Bob also was concerned about losing his penis and spent a good deal of time nude before the mirror, ap-

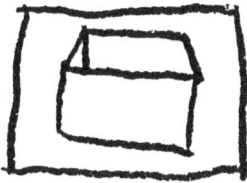

Fig. 5

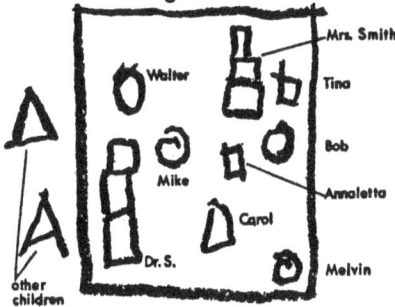

Fig. 6 ▲ Children's Group

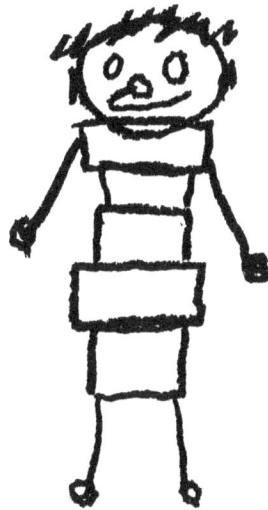

Fig. 7

parently making sure it was still there. The most fascinating examples of problems relating to the body image, and evidence of its extreme fragility, occurred during the trips to the large swimming pool. Here we noticed that Bob was clutching his penis and would not look down into the water. We had to give detailed and elaborate explanations to assure him that his body was still there even when he could not see it under water. Similarly, the children at the pool-side seemed terrified at the perception of heads without visibly attached bodies, apparently floating on the surface. We felt that our interpretations were correct because reassurances based on them did greatly allay the children's anxiety.

Early in therapy, Mike and Walter displayed a remarkable facility to control affect and impulsive action, but only on an "all-or-none" basis. They gave no evidence of having impulses to play with toys, to explore the new area, to inspect the new people in the environment, nor even to eat and drink. Their "dead-pan" expressions revealed no evidence of feeling joy or pleasure, pain or sadness, or ordinary anger. They never laughed or cried; impulse and affect were released only in their explosive episodes of rage. Tina sat expressionless and immobile except when mouthing a wire or shoelace, at which time she seemed to anticipate a struggle to remove it from her mouth. Bob, in spite of all his provocative exhibitionistic behavior, revealed no external expressions indicating that he was feeling emotions. Annaletta similarly showed no facial signs of anger, joy, fear or the like—only an anxious, expectant attitude. We felt the control of impulse and affect to be part of the magical control of all stimuli which was used to exclude reality and maintain the desired symbiosis. Autistic defenses therefore were seen to include control or denial of not only external, but also internal stimuli.

After penetration of the autistic defenses and subsidence of the panicky rage-like reactions, impulse control became the responsibility of the therapist. The ultimately safe therapeutic symbiosis permitted the children to act in limited ways which gradually included play with toys, exploration of the surroundings and of their own and others' bodies, and to follow impulses to eat or drink. Their highly aggressive urges were directed into harmless activities such as hitting the inflated clown or "kicking the wall instead." When the therapists were quite certain that a particular affect was being felt by the child or the group, the affect was named. The therapists also verbalized their own feelings where pertinent.

We have stated that most of the activity in the early months of therapy was understood in terms of the child's need to maintain the symbiosis. Actions which the parents usually called "misbehavior" seemed in fact to be intended to gain physical interaction with the therapist. Presumably such behavior at home did lead reliably to contact with the parents. Examples are Tina's mouthing inedible objects and licking walls, Bob's perseverative questioning and turning lights on and off, Mike's exhibitionistic utterances and display of his penis,

Walter's throwing toys, and Annaletta's spitting on the floor or prancing about nude. Although the children displayed little or no affect with these behaviorisms, all the therapists felt the children expected them to be angry or to have some emotional reaction. It was as if action came from the child and affect from the mother, the child's actions being calculated to evoke the desired affect and thus to verify the continued existence of the symbiosis. Hence we believed that such actions of the children were part of their magical, manipulative patterns for maintaining symbiosis. Autistic activity with its hallucinatory potential, fetishistic behavior with a "thing," and misbehavior aimed at producing a specific response in the mother, all of these in effect reconstituted the symbiosis.

As therapy progressed and the group symbiosis became "safer," it became possible for the children to be more active, to perceive and heed impulses to explore the surroundings, other people, and their own bodies. Concurrently, the children began to show visible evidence of various feelings and ultimately exhibited appropriate expressions of joy and pleasure (including childish laughter), pain and sadness (with real tears), and appropriate and controllable anger, jealously, rivalry, and envy.

Our ideas of the nature of the psychotic child's sense of personal identity are at the outset highly speculative, since visible evidence of its existence is conspicuously absent. Infantile global omnipotence is not conducive to a sense of identity, since it *includes* everything and does not distinguish self from world. Regressive autism might seem the converse, but since it *excludes* everything, there is nothing left to distinguish the self *from*. In fact, recognition of Self is impossible without simultaneous recognition of Other. The word "identity" comes from "idem," meaning "the same," implying "same as self" (integrity, persistence), and "different from others" (uniqueness, separateness). We would guess that in the psychotic child there is some primitive self-awareness, more

visceral than intellectual, or reactivity to hungers and grati-
fications, but no awareness of self as a perceptive being. This
"pre-identity" may include recollection of the repetitive interactions with the real or fantasied mother, later controlled by
the child, but it is possible that no real distinction is made
between a current interaction and a past one. However, once
the safe group symbiosis was accepted in which the boundaries
of the group were progressively delineated, a body image
gradually defined, and ways of coping with impulse and affect
developed, we saw evidence of the growth of a definite interest
in people, and with it, manifestations of the development of a
real identity.

When the children first developed communicative speech,
they did not use "I" or "me" in referring to themselves, but
rather "you": "You want to go to the bathroom," etc., often
with a rising inflection which made it sound like a question.
Presumably this was mimicking the parental tone of voice,
where such statements made about the child often *are* questions. Later self-references made use of the child's name: Bob
stopped saying "you" and would say "Bob want to go to the
bathroom." By the end of the second year of therapy all the
children were using pronouns correctly.

The group interactions demonstrated steps in the children's
development of identity. Much of the early looking at, touching, or even struggling with another child seemed to be ex-
ploratory in nature, as if aimed at comprehending this odd
facet of the outside world. We speculate that at first each
child recognized the similarity of the other children, but probably had no clear idea that he, too, was like them. Mike's
statement that "all children have anuses" thus related not only
to his castration anxiety but also the recognition that he was a
child like the others. The concern about girls, and close inspection of them, was a second step, encompassing simultaneous similarity and difference, as if to say "We are alike
in being small and being called children, but there are two

kinds of children, one kind with a penis and one kind without." This seemed to coincide with a diminution of anxiety about loss of self through engulfment or merging with others. It is as if when names were given to parts and to people, a trend emerged, an *abstract* trend. The individual child can identify (be identical) with *the abstract idea of a child,* while his relation to the parts of other children he gradually realizes to be *similarity,* and not identity. True identity means "you and I are one and the same, there is only one person here." Similarity means "you and I meet the criteria of the abstraction 'a child,' but we are separate and the relation is likeness and not sameness." Perhaps some of the early behavior in front of the mirror can be used to illustrate this point: when a child approached the mirror, the image *was* the same, in that "the other" corresponded not only in appearance but also in movement; this meant it was also under control of the child and in some ways approximated his feelings of magical control of the symbiosis. However, when he noted the other children via the mirror, not responding to his magical control, it was like mother not responding to the proper cues. When the abstraction "children" emerges, then neither similarity nor difference are threatening. It was early in the third year of therapy before the children became aware of yet another level of mutual similarity, namely parents, and in particular mothers. This added realm of "things in common" then extended to talk of grandparents, aunts, and uncles.

The sense of personal identity was however always tenuous. For instance, when Annaletta put on Bob's shoes, Bob asked, "Who is Annaletta now?" Clothes were included in the body image, and the children were all concerned about leaving their bathing suits in the therapy room, as though leaving part of themselves behind, with consequent alteration of identity. The change from long pants to shorts occasioned similar concern and questions. Mike feels he would lose his identity if he complied with an adult's request, which makes control and communication difficult. He seems to be in constant conflict over his wish to merge with his mother *vs.* his wish for individuation. This presents a problem in the school setting, as he seems to feel that if he does what the teacher asks, he would no longer be Mike. This attitude creates hazards for the teacher, as it is all too easily seen as simple stubbornness.

Of the four aspects of ego we have discussed, we believe the sense of personal identity to be the most fragile. It develops in the face of a constant wish to merge with the mother in a permanent symbiosis. Therapy fosters the development of identity, which has its own appeal to the psychotic ego, but the two tendencies are opposed and, metaphorically speaking, they struggle for dominance. The therapists constantly thwart maneuvers toward symbiosis and try to make identity stronger and tolerable, but the child's frustration tolerance is low and his ambivalence intense. At the same time the mother also has strong unconscious wishes to maintain the symbiotic state.

THE MOTHER: BAD CHILD VS. GOOD MOTHER

The mother's contribution to the pathological symbiosis is reconstructed from data obtained from the mothers' group therapy. Each mother expected the unborn child to make up for a lifetime of frustrated hopes and longings. The group clearly stated this anticipation when they spoke of marriage, the birth of the now psychotic child, and the beginning of therapy as being similar in that each was anticipated as fulfilling lifelong goals. Mrs. W. vividly stated her expectations of the child when she wrote: "In his perfection, my imperfections will disappear." Similarly, Bob's birth was to restore the bliss of the early years of marriage for Mrs. B., and equally fantastic expectations of Tina and Mike could be inferred from the mother's verbalizations during group therapy. The failure of the child to fulfill these egocentric wishes dealt each mother a profound narcissistic wound. To every action of the child which failed to gratify her fantasy, the mother reacted as though accused of being a "bad mother" or an inferior, despicable person (the "bad self"). She then made frantic, angry attempts to coerce the child to act "right." If the child responded correctly to this manipulation, she then felt, "I am a good mother, a good person." It was consistently evident that most of the mother's acts toward the child were motivated out of needs arising in herself and rarely as a result of maternal responses to the child's communications of his own needs. Since the child's actual needs were not met, he of course did not respond positively, and consequently the mother experienced her interaction with the child as an accusation of bad mothering rather than a confirmation of good mothering ability. She felt that the child purposely bedeviled her, and she wanted help in understanding the child's actions so that she could make him behave properly. We felt that "behave properly" really meant "make mother feel good."

This interaction between mother and child was evident in all the child's activities and in every phase of development, in feeding and sleeping, diapering and bowel training, speech and learning, and the development of "manners." It seems clear that with such inappropriate maternal expectations, we need not postulate innate biological or anatomical defects (such as might prohibit normal responses by the child) in order to account for pathological mother-child interactions. On the other hand, the existence of any such defect in the child would almost certainly accentuate the mother's disappointment and her tendency to disparage her competence as a mother and a person, which would in turn increase her need to control and manipulate the child to make him act and be "right."

Throughout therapy, all the mothers persistently clung to their need to disavow, deny, or somehow get rid of all wishes, impulses, and feelings which they designated as "bad." Mrs. B. and Mrs. M. clung to their "perfect" ego ideal right up to the final session, and considered the termination of therapy to be a rejection of them and a demand that they rid themselves of whatever "badness" remained. Mrs. T. refused to accept the group's allegation of her "badness," projected it onto her husband, and steadfastly refused to alter her behavior unless the husband changed. Mrs. W. also denied the implication of the group that she was "bad" and merely designated her demands as the rights of one who has suffered such deprivation. Mrs. A. persistently condemned the bad behavior of Annaletta (and the badness of others who constantly involved her with the law) and presented herself as a distraught but co-operative mother, who did her best to do the right thing for her sick child, and who was innocently entangled in the irresponsible behavior of others. We translated these attitudes as meaning that the mothers felt that their children were primarily expected to behave in such a way as to demonstrate the mothers' "goodness," and hence to prove the absence of "badness."

Such an attitude does not by itself constitute or cause a pathological symbiosis. The mother's unrealistic expectations of the child and her consequent narcissistic hurt are only the first steps in this direction. The second step involves reactivation of the mother's traumatic and conflictual symbiotic experience with her own mother. All these women as young children had been involved in a non-psychotic but unsatisfactory symbiotic relationship with their mothers, and then suffered the trauma of having mother abruptly turn away from them, in many instances due to the birth of a sibling. They seem to have ascribed this tragedy to their own "badness," especially the "badness" of infantile instinctual demands. They dealt with their bruised instincts in a variety of ways, but all were left with profound unconscious needs to become a "good child" in order to regain and hold the mother's love. Many, subsequently, had normal children, and presumably had performed normal mothering. But at the birth of the children who are now our patients, it happened that old repressed, unintegrated instincts and feelings were aroused which brought back the terrible old feeling of "badness." Integration being impossible, a desperate solution was achieved by radical splitting of "goodness" and "badness" into "good mother" and "good child," "bad mother" and "bad child." The mothers restored themselves to "goodness" by ascribing *all* "badness" to the "bad, sick child," including not only the child's normally arising infantile demands, but the mother's old hostility, envy, etc., regardless of how remote its cause or recent re-arousal. In such a situation, past and present are undistinguishable, and the mother and child become inseparable. The mother's unresolved symbiosis of the past is reconstituted in the present, and in the present mother-child symbiosis, she acts out her struggle to regain the blissful symbiosis of the real or fancied past. At the same time, the mother's internal struggle against badness is externalized and dealt with in the manipulative interaction between mother and child.

In the mothers' group therapy the group transference was one of an "all good child" being fed by an "all good mother." All "badness" was rejected, denied, or projected. Mrs. W., T., and M. related to the group therapist as if he were the source of all knowledge and understanding; Mrs. B., on the other hand, saw him as a persecutor. The first three saw "all other people" as incompetent, inadequate, and undesirable, while Mrs. B's "perfect person" was "taller than the therapist." They all envisioned the group (the "good child") relating to the therapist (the "good mother") as a never-ending state of bliss. All undesirable events, including interpretive remarks made by the therapist, were treated as threatening disruptions and were excluded as rapidly as possible. Sexuality was seen by the group as the greatest threat to the constancy of the blissful symbiosis and was vigorously excluded by the group for over two years. Hence all sexual impulses (both infantile and mature) were vigorously repressed, suppressed, denied, or projected as potential threats to the group symbiosis. Similarly, infantile sexual impulses in the children were vigorously attacked by the mothers. Interruption of the symbiosis was equated with death, which may account for the tenacity with which the mothers clung to the symbiosis in therapy and the real-life symbiotic relationship with the child.

NEUROTIC FAMILY INTERACTION

Our understanding of the interaction within these families was derived from several sources: chiefly from material revealed in the parents' therapy groups and from reconstructive correlation of behavior observed in the parents' and children's groups. There were many direct glimpses of family interaction, but no systematic observation. In particular, the beginning and end of the children's sessions afforded many opportunities for brief glimpses of mother and child under the stress of parting. Occasional joint meetings of the parents' groups were held. There were no formal observations of total family groups, but on two occasions all the parents and children attended a Christmas party, and one of these the normal siblings attended also.

To a superficial view, these families presented a picture of conservative middle-class respectability in which both parents functioned in a socially adequate manner. Each mother seemed to think of herself (and was viewed by the community) as intelligent, socially competent, and perhaps more than adequate as a mother, harrassed and made miserable by a peculiar, obnoxious child. Each father was seen as a bright, competent, responsible family man who properly fulfilled his role in the community. The parents clung tenaciously to this façade and defended it with great energy.

Close beneath this thin veneer of socially acceptable, culturally designated role-fulfillment were seriously neurotic patterns of interaction. The fathers of these children are best described as absent psychologically, and were in some cases physically absent. Their unavailability left the mother without support of her emotional needs, the son without object for identification, and the daughter unable to gain feelings of acceptance. Actually the typical father competes with the child for the mother's attention. In the structured, male-oriented world of business and profession, the husband performs adequately, but in the home his role identification seems blurred and confusing, and he is anxious. At times he is hypermasculine and authoritarian, at other times passive and childlike. He seeks reassurance of his adequacy as a man, and although he gains verbal praise from his wife, she also behaves in ways which effectively emasculate him. Similarly, the husband verbally reassures his wife of her adequacy as a woman, but by his behavior depreciates and maligns the feminine role.

Communication between husband and wife was confined to trivial matters in order to avoid expression of the profound feelings of frustration and anger which each felt toward the other. We feel that the father abdicated in favor of the mother-child unit to avoid the necessity of coping with his wife's emotional needs and demands. When his own need to be mothered became urgent, he actively competed with the child and attempted to push the child aside long enough to gain gratification of his own wishes. He would then retreat and permit mother and child to reunite.

The mothers' attempts to maintain social approval and a façade of proper role identity barely hid inner feelings of intense frustration, low self-esteem, and nearly uncontrollable rage. Deeply mistrusting their spontaneous emotional responses, these women relied on superficial but rigid ideas of how nice, normal husbands and wives are "supposed" to feel in all situations, and they adhered faithfully to these notions, regardless of what their actual feelings might be. "Good" and "bad" were sharply separated, all "goodness" ascribed to the parents and any "badness" relegated to the child. The mothers dealt with imperfections of character or behavior in themselves and their husbands by denial, rationalization, for-giveness, or "acceptance" at an intellectual level, although they did not in fact understand emotionally that these imperfec-tions are simply inevitable human characteristics. On the other hand, most infantile behavior such as crying, irritability, impatience, fear, and frustration was seen as reprehensible and totally unacceptable.

The mother's interaction with the child was reminiscent of a little girl playing with her doll, where she plays the role of an idealized mother who takes complete care of the child; at the same time, she identifies herself with the "baby" who is mothered. The little girl is in complete control—the doll has no feelings or motivations beyond what the "mother" attributes to it. She projects her good self onto the doll, amiably enjoying the rewarding interchange of good mother and good child. The little girl in addition projects her own capacity for bad-ness onto the doll at times and must then punish it to drive away the badness.

With the psychotic children, their mothers seem to have reverted to this latency-type of mothering, particularly with respect to the mother's attribution to the child of her own needs or feelings. The child is engaged in some activity, and the mother suddenly goes to him and covers him with hugs and kisses, quite without regard to his own wishes of the moment. We saw this often as the children were assembling for therapy sessions, where the mother's actual need may have been to display active motherly behavior, however inappropriate this may have been at the time. Alternatively, the mother may sud-denly expect the child to perform in some manner or other and become very angry if he does not respond to her wish (or, alternatively, if the wish is for "bad" behavior, become angry if he *does* respond). Bob had not fiddled with light-switches for weeks, but one day when his mother came to pick him up after therapy, she upbraided him furiously because of her suspicion that he would flip the switches in the halls as he left the clinic; needless to say, Bob flipped them that day. Our therapy room was unusually cool one winter day, and Mike had on a thin sweater when his mother brought him to the room, while she wore a heavy winter coat. After being in the room for five minutes, she dashed to Mike and removed his sweater, stating that he was too hot. It seems more likely that *she* was too hot.

The basic psychological interaction between mother and child was one in which the child's failure to perform according to the mother's needs and expectations seriously threatened her self-concept. The mother's typical response was to attack (perhaps "counter-attack") this threatening child. It was as if the mother and child experienced a gratifying interaction only when the child's response, more or less by chance, coincided with the mother's conscious and unconscious fantasy of the moment. The possibility of such a coincidence was small, because the mother's unconscious wish was quite often directly in opposition to her idealized conscious wish. Indeed, it was rarely that the child could respond "right." It was our impression that the child invariably responded to the mother's unconscious command, to which her conscious wishes, identical to society's oversimplified rational demands, were strongly opposed. She, of course felt righteous indignation at the child's misbehavior and apparently inappropriate responses, and readily obtained the sympathy of friends and neighbors. She was also able to enlist the support of the father in criticizing and punishing the child for his misbehavior.

Although the fathers dimly recognized the contradictoriness of the situation, each could only agree with his wife in her assessment of the child's badness. In most instances it seemed that the father attempted to relate to the child, but found himself also quite incapable of appropriate interaction. We believe that the child attempted to seek normal interaction with the father in an effort to escape the engulfing mother, but the father's psychological remoteness plus his feelings of revulsion toward the child made a relationship between them impossible. Most of the fathers spoke of how some of the child's behavior reminded them of unacceptable aspects of themselves as children, from which they retreated.

There is little question that the parents of these children wanted help in altering the family interaction that was so energy-consuming and so distressing to all. The mothers in particular wished to free themselves from the intense inter-action with the child and wished the child to mature and be-come independent. We attempted to accomplish this change by utilizing the "mammy" to relieve the mother from the intense interaction during the daytime hours, and by providing the mothers with a group therapy experience in which under-standing and support could be given.

The chief problem in the mothers' therapy was that of re-integrating "badness" into the mother's personality. We believe that whatever the mother's total contribution to the child's psychosis may be, her inability to integrate her own infantile impulses is basic. Her ability to project these infantile impulses onto others, including the child, is a lifelong pattern, and represents a fundamental personality defect. This formulation in no way denies the importance of the child's contribution to the perpetuation of this symbiotic interaction. The child's pat-terned experiences and his need to preserve the symbiosis re-quire that he perpetuate the patterned responses in the mother, and there is no denying his adeptness in doing just that. He seems quite willing to pay the price of ridicule, scolding, and assault, provided he can maintain the symbiosis.

It is our belief that the efficacy of therapy, not only of the child, but of the entire family, depends upon the possibility of effecting separation of mother and child, and enabling the mother to integrate her own infantile impulses and to deal with them at a conscious level. It is also essential to assist the father to become available emotionally to the mother, offering an alternative (and more appropriate) source of human relationship. The work with the child helps him to develop an identity which is capable of resisting the tendency to merge with the mother under ordinary conditions of stress. We believe that this identity, once developed, can best be strengthened by utilizing the child's intellectual capacities as a defense against regression in ordinary stressful situations. The group educational program which began during the third year of therapy had this specific goal of utilizing the child's intelligence to further separation-individuation and thus strengthen and stabilize his identity.

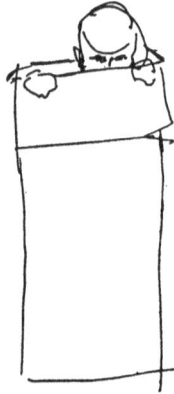

IX · Later Stages of Therapy

During the third year of therapy, the children's group consisted of Mike, Walter, Bob, Tina, Annaletta, Melvin, and
Carol. Walter, by his crayoning, had completed a series of
drawings illustrating the development of a self-identity, the
fact of a "group ego" and his recognition that the group, by
having "group sessions," were different from "other children."
(See p. 132.) Walter initially crayoned in a compulsive to-
and-fro manner without regard to margins. He later drew a
border on each sheet of paper and compulsively remained
within this boundary, becoming very upset if his crayon went
beyond it. He then drew a circle in the center and added
structures which he designated as arms, legs, eyes, and mouth,
but all inside the circle, which was in turn within the boundary
lines. Walter later attempted to draw houses but had great
difficulty with the perspective of the roof and once again
experienced anxiety when he was unable to do this drawing
correctly or if his lines went beyond the borders he had drawn.
Once he had mastered the house outline, he made his rounded
figures inside the house, and designated them collectively as

"the children's group." He drew figures of a different shape outside the house, and called them "other children." He finally drew several squares on top of one another, made a circle at the top, and added arms and legs in appropriate places, along with eyes, ears, hair, and mouth. His final addition was feet on the legs and hands on the arms.

That this newfound identity was fragile is indicated by the questions the children asked. For instance, if Annaletta put on Bob's shoes, Bob wanted to know "Who is Annaletta now?" Similarly, if Annaletta removed her dress and played in her panties, Bob became quite anxious, took off all his clothing, paraded before the mirror and expressed his concern that he was no longer Bob. The children were quite worried about leaving their bathing suits in the group room, and it was only after several such expressions of anxiety that we concluded they feared a loss of identity should they go home without their swim suits. When this was discussed with them, they brought forth some more concerns about changing from short pants to long pants; all this was related to concerns about loss of identity. We had a great deal of difficulty in dealing with body image anxiety when we took the children swimming. We noted that those on the edge of the pool were upset, but quite fascinated, by observing the children in the water up to their necks. It was necessary to have the child come out of the water and demonstrate that he was not really bodiless, in order to allay the anxiety. Similarly, the child in the water was unable to observe his own body under the water because of the optical distortion. We found Bob intent on holding his head and eyes upward and refusing to look down, but grasping his penis with his hands all the while. We had to have him look at our bodies in the water and to tell him that it was the same body that was outside the water, that the body did not actually change. In addition to anxieties about identity and bodily integrity, concerns about total destruction, castration, and sexual differences appeared repeatedly in the group therapy.

Four of the children had attended a kindergarten during the second year of therapy and were able to adapt to a tolerable degree. At the beginning of the third year all were evidencing a keen interest in the real world and seemed most at ease when the situation was relatively well structured. Bob, Walter, Mike, and Annaletta frequently asked to be shown how to read and write and seemed gratified when they could reproduce certain letters and numbers. We concluded that the children were ready for some preschool training and accordingly, designated a certain portion of each session as "school time" and secured the services of two special education teachers. Each session was begun with a short, unstructured period wherein initial exuberance and anxiety could be expressed. Then "school time" was announced, small chairs were lined up in front of the blackboard, and the teacher was introduced to the group. She shook hands with each child, and in so doing distinguished right from left hand. She also made a distinction between boys and girls by having the boys stand up to shake hands, while the girls remained seated. The children began work by learning to write their names, writing numbers, and naming colors. We soon learned the necessity for exact replication in each session in order to avoid confusing the children; every letter and number had to be done exactly the same way each time. Difficulty in transposing from the blackboard to paper was frequently encountered and could only be overcome by repetition and explanation. Problems were also presented by the left-handedness of Mike, Walter, and Bob. We solved this by having the teacher stand behind the child when showing him how to print on the blackboard. Bob had a strong tendency to write backwards, especially when printing his name. He was finally able to communicate his dislike of himself and his wish to avoid seeing "himself" in print.

The teachers were sorely tried by Mike's refusal to follow directions. He clearly knew what was being asked of him, and also seemed to want to comply. We learned that on the way home from the sessions, he repeated the entire exercise, exactly as requested by the teacher. In the classroom, however, he managed to destroy almost every paper or other work he was requested to do. He always did this destructive act in an exhibitionistic and silly way (for instance, he might put several lines on the "E"). We wondered why he needed to appear stupid and told him we knew that he could do what the teacher asked. We ultimately recognized Mike's need to be autonomous in his performance. It was as if he so feared losing his fragile identity that he was unable to comply with another's request, as though compliance would indicate he was no longer Mike. The ultimate in this negativism appeared when he drew beachballs rather than do the prescribed assignment. We dealt with the situation by interpretation and by granting him permission to be himself; instead of *telling* him what to do, we suggested he *might* do some task if he wished. Mike's work is very good and he evidently has above-average intelligence, but if complimented on his performance, he will refuse to go on, as though simply pleasing another person might be as dangerous as compliance. When Mike entered regular school, this behavior was difficult for his teacher to cope with and she responded by an oversolicitous attitude which alienated Mike even further. Once she was able to comprehend the situation and to leave him alone, his work was excellent. During the third year of therapy, Mike learned to read, write, and do simple arithmetic, but his attitude toward authority figures remained negativistic. We encountered great difficulty in persuading his mother to refrain from insisting that he act according to her wishes. When he failed to be promoted from the first to the second grade, his mother called him an "irresponsible baby" and then made unreasonable demands on him. Following this, his performance in the group was one of complying with the label "irresponsible baby," but if given complete attention by a therapist, he behaved like the usual schoolboy.

Bob's tendency to reading reversal and mirror-writing hampered early reading and writing. However, once he had developed better self-esteem he gave convincing proof of his ability to learn. His first experience in public school, however, was catastrophic. His mother was quite unable to tolerate the separation and became increasingly anxious as the days passed. On the tenth day she went to his teacher and questioned her closely about whether Bob had been misbehaving, as she feared. His anxiety increased and very soon he began acting as his mother had expected. When he found some paint and painted a drinking fountain, he was immediately expelled from school, permanently. The parents responded by markedly depreciating Bob and expressing great hostility towards the therapist (RWS). They began a desperate search for another school and, without consulting us, enrolled him in a private first grade. This lasted less than two weeks, and by the time the private school teachers requested consultation with the therapist, the situation had deteriorated beyond repair. At this point Bob began working with a tutor, and his learning rapidly increased, to the satisfaction of both himself and his mother. We were able to use these events to illustrate to the mother her own reactions to separation and the effect her anxiety has on Bob in such situations. As a result, Bob was able to separate a good deal from his mother and began seeking peer relationships within the treatment group, designating various children as "friend." He was also permitted to explore away from his home and mother and thus experienced separation without excessive anxiety. At the end of the third year, Bob could write well, read moderately well, and do simple arithmetic. He had a long attention span and was capable of responding to most of the teacher's requests.

Walter's impulsive behavior caused considerable difficulty in the school situation. However, his desire to learn was strong, and he seemed eager to understand the material presented. One of the biggest problems was his frustration whenever he was unable to reproduce a letter, number, or drawing. He per-severed, however, and learned to print numbers and letters and read simple words. When using flash cards for vocabulary testing, we were surprised at his ability to read many words that we had not known he understood. It was often noted that he remained fixated on certain colors or words, and espe-cially the figures 9, 10, and 11 on the clock which had been used to teach the children time concepts. Walter was often impatient and tended to grab whatever material was offered and to use it as he saw fit without waiting for explanations. Walter attended a kindergarten during the second year of therapy and most of the third year. His mother had been afraid to start him in an advanced kindergarten in the first portion of the third year, out of fear that he would disappoint her by failing. This was clearly related to her competitive attitude toward the mothers of Mike and Bob, who were at-tempting a first grade placement for their children. It was only after Bob had failed to remain in the public first grade that Mrs. W. permitted Walter to enter the advanced kindergarten. One of the greatest problems with Walter has been in helping him to differentiate what is acceptable behavior from what is not. It is as though he had been permitted in the home to indulge in all behavior for a period of time, followed by prohibition of all activities when his mother became angry with him. In the therapy sessions we permitted fairly boister-ous behavior during the recess and recreation periods, but insisted on quite controlled behavior during the school period. At the end of the third year of therapy, Walter was able to control himself for periods of 20-30 minutes, during which time he could concentrate on his work. Once the school activity was over, he responded with immediate exuberance which we restrained moderately, making limits most explicit. There was little doubt that Walter was ready for public schooling, al-though we felt the problem of self-control might be taxing to his teacher.

Tina attended a nursery school during the second year of therapy and a kindergarten the third year. There was some initial separation anxiety, but this soon ceased; although Tina was more of a passive observer than an active participant, she remained in the kindergarten setting without undue distress to herself or the teacher. Her younger sister accompanied her the first part of the second year, and this seemed to inhibit Tina's activities to a considerable degree. In the latter part of the third year, at the teacher's request, they were separated, and efforts were made to stimulate Tina into productive activity on her own. In the therapy-education sessions, Tina's productions were limited. We noted that she did the best work when relating one-to-one with an adult. She could not easily concentrate on just one thing and was often distracted by other children or adults in the room. In fact, she seemed to prefer relating to them and as a result withdrew her attention entirely from the teacher and the work. At times her behavior suggested confabulation, in that when she did not know how to answer questions, she would respond irrelevantly, with the facial grimaces and posturing that are so characteristic of her mother's seductive behavior. Some observers felt that Tina was mentally retarded, although psychological testing showed too much spread among subtests to clearly confirm this impression.

Mrs. A. would not permit Annaletta to enter a school until the fall of the third year. On the first day of school Annaletta had a tantrum and the school authorities promptly requested her removal. She was finally placed in an ungraded primary and was able to maintain her composure and to profit from the school experience. She approached learning with remarkable avidity, but still reverted to uttering gibberish whenever she was puzzled or confused. She did, however, learn to count, read some words, and write. She followed instructions quite readily, and gained a good deal of gratification from her productions. The home situation deteriorated markedly in that Mrs. A. was unable to keep out of trouble with the law.

She was in court many times because of disturbances at her home involving her ex-husband and boyfriends. It seems as though once Annaletta had separated from her mother, Mrs. A. could no longer contain her "bad" impulses and began acting on them.

Carol had no experience of schooling outside the therapeutic education program. Her behavior in the sessions was puzzling: when the teacher asked her to print her name, she instead looked at herself in the mirror and seemed to be watching herself perform. If the teacher became insistent, Carol would begin to cry and then go to the mirror to watch herself cry, saying, "She likes to cry"; "She is pretty when she cries"; and "Mother watches her cry." We interpreted this to mean that Carol's relationship with her mother was one in which Carol cries and thus gains mother's attention (at least her visual attention).

Melvin clung tenaciously to his autism and resisted penetration of these defenses for a long period of time. He maintained autistic withdrawal from the adults in the room for over a year, although he was willing to make contact with the other children after some six months of therapy. His autism continued well into his second year of treatment and only during the latter part of the group's third year did he begin to utter sounds and syllables which could be precursors of words. Up to this time his vocal noises were mainly humming, growls, and later sounds of laughter. The question of deafness persisted for many months and only occasionally could we be entirely sure that he was able to hear. In the latter part of the second year of his treatment he formed strong group attachments and mimicked several other children in the group. This was noted especially in his drawing and in the group ritual of shaking hands with the teacher. In front of the mirror he would raise an arm or leg, move his head, or jump about. He was intrigued by motion and often played a game of putting a block on the sill of the mirror, and moving himself from side to side while intently observing the block. He would then take the block in his hand and move it in front of the mirror, holding himself stationary. He then held the block in his hand and moved both himself and the block across the length of the mirror while observing both. We spent a good deal of time with him at the mirror, naming parts of his body and telling him that they belonged to him. We noticed that he kept his mouth shut and would not investigate it with his finger as the other children had done. Later he cautiously inserted his finger between his lips, as though tentatively exploring. The therapist then put his own finger into Melvin's mouth, and told him it was a mouth, and that he could talk with it if he wished. We also offered our own mouths for his inspection. Shortly after this, we heard him for the first time utter consonants. It is apparent that his mother fancies that he is an extension of herself and that she does the talking for him. Much of his head moving and growling sounds are an identification with his father and represent some attempt on his part to individuate. Intensive work with the mother resulted in a considerable degree of separation in the latter part of this period. It was evident that Melvin was clearly interested in our school sessions and when not frightened, he participated actively and co-operatively. He often withdrew from the group suddenly, but could be readily persuaded to return to it. He had a much better relationship with the group than with the adult therapists.

Once the pre-school educational program with its necessary structure was started, group anxiety lessened. We gradually increased the amount of time the children spent in the structured situation and decreased the unstructured time. We had to set limits enough to permit teaching, but at the same time wished to be sufficiently permissive that the children could act out or otherwise display their current conflicts. When home stresses were minimal, the school sessions were quite productive. When family and other environmental stresses were great, the children would be restless and unproductive. But if we attempted to impose significant restrictions when the children were under stress, they often reacted with disruptive behavior which we could neither understand nor interpret because of its explosive nature. At such times we allowed the children to act out and verbalize so that we could "diagnose," interpret, and clarify the conflicts producing the increased anxiety. Invariably, these anxieties related to intense interactions in the home.

In attempting to understand the possibilities of teaching the psychotic children, it was our impression that at first, inanimate things were strongly invested with affects displaced from people, and the therapy was largely directed towards "depersonalizing" these fetishistic objects. Once this had been achieved, and the affects redirected toward people as objects of interest, love, hate, etc., then *learning* about inanimate reality became possible. The teaching program emphasized formal and abstract properties of things, for instance numbers, words, colors, shapes, names, time, and distance, but now without the ambivalent affect which had been present during the psychotic phase. This was not always easy, however, since whenever the child was suffering from conflict, he tended to project and displace the conflict onto something inanimate and then attempt to work it out by excessive fixation on the thing. For instance, whenever Mike began (inappropriately) to draw beachballs, we understood that some conflict was causing him serious distress. If we were aware of what was going on at home, it was often possible to interpret the conflict to him, after which he would be able to relinquish this preoccupation with beachballs and get on with the lesson. Walter often used certain colors (blue and red) in a similar obsessive manner. He drew countless pictures of a Volkswagen, working out his anxiety about an accident involving the family car, and he manifested concerns about the insides of things with his series of drawings of a washing machine. We could not unravel the meaning of his fixation on the numbers 9, 10, and 11 on the clock-face. Bob did not use inanimate objects to assuage his anxiety, but related to people in an obsessive way, getting as close to an adult as possible and asking endless irrelevant questions in a singsong voice.

The goals of early therapy were focused on helping the child to attain separation-individuation and to develop a stable identity. Later, therapy and education worked hand-in-hand in establishing realistic relationships to the world of things. Therapy helped divest objects of their fetishistic taint, by interpretation of underlying conflicts and affects, substituting verbal concepts about the human objects actually involved; education at the same time provided names, properties, and uses for the objects, permitting them to be re-invested with functionally appropriate libido. Learning, in any real sense, is impossible until the child has worked through the conflictual affect fixated on the tangible objects of his world, but when this has been accomplished, his energy is free so that he may engage in egosyntonic learning. The teaching program was of course unavoidably interrupted by the environmental stresses placed on these children, invariably involving an interaction between child and mother. In nearly every instance the interaction involved the basic dynamics wherein the mother's narcissism was wounded and she attacked the child in a misguided effort to force him to "behave right." Certainly the child often provoked such interactions, but we were unable to prevent the mothers from habitually acting in this manner without provocation.

FOURTH YEAR OF CHILDREN'S GROUP

During the fourth year, the problems most often in focus were the conflicts and attendant anxieties of the phallic phase of psychosexual development. Therapy attempted to strengthen what anxiety and regression weakened, in the following areas: (1) Ability to tolerate affect and control impulse. (2) Reality testing ability, intellectual activity and defense mechanisms. (3) Whole-object perception and relationships, and object constancy. (4) Affirmation of self-identity separate from both mother and group. The conflicts were so intense that impulse and affect control were frequently disrupted; regression from more mature defense mechanisms occurred, and attempts were made to return to the symbiotic mode, which had been partially abandoned.

During the period from May to November of the fourth year (1963) tension within the group increased markedly. The teaching program was frequently interrupted by sudden outbursts of boisterous behavior by the boys (not including Bob), and the girls also gave evidence of rising tension. Walter continued to provoke interactions with adults by acting on his aggressive impulses at will and refusing to co-operate in group activities unless he felt like it. Mike seemed sad and desperate. Whenever he failed to perform as she wished, his mother called him an "irresponsible baby," and he seemed bent on proving the accuracy of this label. Melvin related to the group in a playful, affectionate way, but continued to avoid contact with the adults as much as possible. His mother had removed him from the group during the summer months, and it was six weeks before he could wholeheartedly re-enter it. He co-operated only intermittently with the teaching program and took delight in the opportunities for rough-housing with the other boys. Bob appeared more and more passive-feminine as he stepped up his defenses against assuming an aggressive masculine role. He was docile and co-operative, but a master at provoking hostile interactions between others, then immediately withdrawing to a safe position by a teacher or female therapist.

The girls in the group were shy and reluctant to interact with the boys, but remarkably willing to co-operate with the teachers. Shirley and Darlene, the new members, soon became an integral part of the group, although they were initially greeted by assaults on the part of the boys. Carol continued to jabber her irrelevant phrases, cried a good deal, and spent a lot of time observing herself in the mirror. When asked to do something, she promptly cried and insisted that she had to go to the bathroom. She was a frequent target for male aggression, since she reacted so quickly and impressively to even a gestural threat of attack. Tina stood her ground with the boys and frequently ridiculed them. For instance, when Mike stood on the table, dropped his trousers and urinated in a high arc to the floor, Tina said, "I can do that too, but *I* do it in the toilet." When pressed to reveal her comprehension of a day's lesson, Tina usually reverted to silly behavior, such as insisting that she was a cat or dog. She was an accomplished flirt and spent much time trying to manipulate the therapists and teachers with her coyness. Annaletta's attendance was very irregular, and in the late fall her mother withdrew her from treatment, saying that it was impossible to bring her any longer. Mrs. A.'s involvement with the community authorities became increasingly complex, and her home life so chaotic that Annaletta's state of neglect came to the attention of her school; the Welfare Department was given custody by the Court, and Anna was placed in a foster home.

In the spring of 1963, the routine was as follows: at the start of each session the group was permitted to "blow off steam" for a brief period, and then regular school activities were held for 30-35 minutes. Then there was a 20-minute recess in the yard outside, or in the gym if the weather was bad. Returning to the group room, the children had cookies and milk, and then a final 30-minute handcrafts session. But gradually the opening period of exuberance increased in length, and it became increasingly difficult to get the children to change over to the structured teaching period. The boys interacted aggressively, attacked the girls, and appeared to be inviting each other to "act up." Darlene behaved quite seductively, especially toward Mike, who would frequently lash out at her, spit on her, and grab at her genitals. Sometimes he threw her to the floor and made copulatory movements. Later he exposed his penis and succeeded in urinating on her. Although she responded to all this with tears and demands for adult protection, the observers noted that she persisted in acting seductively toward Mike. Whenever tension mounted, but without behavioral discharge, Bob would manage to precipitate some action by doing something to get Mike and Walter tussling together. Walter became more and more active and managed to disrupt many sessions with his aggressive behavior, which seemed more manipulative than hostile. The boys became increasingly exhibitionistic and commonly urinated on the floor. Each such act was fraught with anxiety, to which the entire group responded. Usually this anxiety-driven behavior included an attack on the girls, and finally a rather vicious struggle between two of the boys.

In December the staff recognized the futility of continuing the formal teaching program until the anxiety and fantasies underlying this wild behavior could be dealt with psychotherapeutically. In order to allow the therapists and observers to understand the conflicts and help the children with them, we "took the lid off" and allowed the group to act out their fantasies without limit of time.

The immediate response was a vigorous display of phallic concerns. Mike seemed determined to prove to all that he had the largest penis in the land and could urinate higher and farther than anyone else. He disrobed completely, paraded before the mirror and the girls, demonstrating, and when he ran out of urine, he spat instead. Although Walter hesitated to initiate any such activity, he soon joined forces with Mike, and the two competed fiercely. Bob identified with the girls, and cowered behind the women's skirts. Fortunately, the taunts of Walker and Mike led Bob to make some tentative steps toward identifying with the males in the group, and ultimately he disrobed, displayed his penis, and boasted of his masculine prowess, standing on a table and urinating as far as Mike. This identification was not without anxiety, however, and he frequently returned to the feminine attitude. He delighted in seeing Mike and Walter act out and frequently provoked them into such behavior. He also wanted the girls to remove their panties and show themselves off, but was unable to get any of them to comply. Carol seemed the most resistant to reveal her lack of a penis, and we suspected that she was stoutly maintaining a fantasy of possessing one. Tina insisted that being a girl and having no penis was of no consequence; in addition, she pointed with pride to her refined bathroom manners. Shirley giggled and obviously enjoyed the display, while Darlene revealed her excitement by her mock distress. When Annaletta was present, she behaved like Tina and ridiculed the boys' activities. She frequently ignored them and tried to gain everyone's attention in re-enacting traumatic scenes she had witnessed at home; she had seen one of her mother's boyfriends knifing another, and had probably been exposed to numerous sexual scenes. She frequently played dead or else reverted to her long-abandoned technique of fascination.

We attempted to learn the fantasies of the group and the individual children, but this was often impossible; the anxiety was so great as to permit only action. At the height of this activity, it became customary for a therapist to take the most boisterous boy into the bathroom, to separate him from the stimulation of the group and give him a chance to calm down. Darlene pleaded with the male therapist to take her in there, too. We could not discover what her fantasies were about what went on in the bathroom, but her behavior indicated sexual excitement and anticipation. Bob verbalized fantasies that the boys were being castrated. We often heard phrases such as "Big penis," "Girls don't have a penis," "Pee-pee on you," and "Poo-poo on you." Mike, Walter, and Bob often had erections and spent long periods of time masturbating in front of the mirror. Melvin was excited about all this, and though he refused to participate, seemed to enjoy it vicariously and often provoked activity of this sort in the group.

During one period of tension-filled quiet, the group was enjoying cookies and milk. Mike and Walter had made taunting remarks to one another, but there was no overt action. Bob seemed especially tense and finally poured milk down the front of Darlene's dress. Mike immediately pulled out his penis and urinated on Walter, and Walter quickly returned the compliment. Mike seemed amazed, and reacted as if he had been turned into a girl by this act. He angrily attacked Darlene, kicking and flailing away at her. When he was restrained, he began to spit at Walter. The two then chased each other round and round one of the therapists, each trying to urinate on the other. To the observers it seemed as if each was trying to prove himself the male and the other the female. At this point Mike talked about whether boys could have babies or not. Walter then attacked Bob by spitting and urinating at him. Bob panicked, tore off his clothes, and stood in front of the mirror inspecting his penis.

Behavior like this was repeated at each session for several weeks. The teaching and crafts programs were suspended, and we tried to reduce the level of anxiety by discussing the apparent fantasies, such as: competitive feelings about the size of the penis, with reference both to other boys and to the father; the permanency of the penis; wishes to be a girl and have babies; spitting and urination as substitutes for grown-up sexual behavior; voyeuristic impulses toward the girls; concern about the girls' lack of a penis; fears of growing up, as well as the wish to become a small child again. We told Mike that he responded to Darlene's behavior because it reminded him of some of his mother's actions. Similarly, we confronted Bob with his anxieties about being a boy and asked why it was that he preferred being a girl. He always said that he wanted to be just like his sister and had no desire to be Bob.

The problem for the therapists in coping with this behavior centered around deciding when was the optimum time to interfere and what was the best role to take, whether as external superego (setting limits), or as auxiliary ego when the anxiety became excessive and regressive behavior supervened, with loss of reality testing. The therapists attempted to get the group as a whole, and the individual children, to establish their own limits to this behavior. They were told that it was up to the group to stop behaving this way, and although the therapists would not let anyone be hurt, the group itself had to set and enforce its own limits. When they were ready, they could ask for the teachers to enter, and school would begin. The girls wanted school immediately, and so did Bob. Mike and Walter were less willing to give up the exciting behavior, but even they fairly often said, "Let's have school now." Quite often wildness would break out again after school had begun, and the equipment had to be removed so that the children could act out some more. Learning seemed to proceed rapidly on days when the conflicts had been acted out to the point of exhaustion, but they did not learn much when more than one child was still anxious.

One day Walter terminated the acting-out by announcing, "I am not going to do that any more, and you can't make me." Although the whole group seemed determined to force him to resume his aggressive phallic role, he was adamant and insisted that school should begin. At that point he brought into the room his "Mr. Rabbit," a toy which had been his constant companion at home and school. He said he was sure the children would destroy Mr. Rabbit, yet he deliberately brought him into the room, provoked attacks upon him by the others, and then defended him bravely. (Recall that Walter's "psychotic fetish" [24] had been destroyed by the children in the earliest months of therapy). Eventually the group stopped attacking Mr. Rabbit, and from then Walter called his toy "Miss

24. M. Sperling (1963), Fetishism in children, *Psychoanalytic Quarterly*, 32:374–392.

Rabbit." From that time on, Walter was a model of self-control. Although still very much a boy, he was able to cope with his impulses without particular anxiety or stress. Concomitantly, his communicative speech improved, and he became more positively interested in learning. He no longer tried to provoke attacks upon his toy, and the other children accepted the presence of the rabbit as a matter of course. A similar thing occured in Walter's school when he introduced the rabbit into the classroom and reading circle; he would read for himself and for the rabbit, in different voices; here, too, the other children accepted this companion without demur.

For a long time, if a child was absent from the group, the others would comment on his absence and its possible cause, etc., and often one would imitate his voice and characteristic remarks, perhaps to magically fill up the gap in the group caused by his absence. This eerily accurate mimicry was now also used in the child's presence, to evoke desired or characteristic behavior, particularly aggression. (Indeed, it almost universally makes people angry to be mocked; it is like having someone tamper with your identity). When Walter became "civilized," Mike or Bob often used this device to try to get him to play his former aggressive role. Failing that, one of them might pretend to *be* Walter, and then behave aggressively, magically restoring the missing "aggressive Walter" to the group. Bob's inability to provoke Walter caused him much anxiety, as if he must soberly accept the responsibility for his own aggressive wishes, now that he could no longer get others to act them out for him. Recall that Bob had slyly acted out his mother's unconscious destructive wishes, and her earliest complaints of "knowing" what horrid things he would do in a store or a friend's home. Bob relinquished much of his feminine manner and at least partially accepted the masculine aggressive role during this period, but still stated verbally that he wished to be a girl. Melvin seemed to thrive on all the excitement, and responded avidly to the educational program.

When his mother removed him from the treatment for the summer (as was her wont) he was just beginning to whisper into the teacher's ear and consistently pointed to written words which related to talking. The girls were acting very much like ordinary little girls, but not in an age-appropriate way.

Mike fared rather badly in all this. The repeated frustration of his omnipotent phallic wishes resulted in intense feelings of worthlessness, and he displayed exceedingly sad affect. He talked incessantly of badness, dying, falling off fire escapes, and lying down in front of cars. He seemed to be constantly testing his lovableness in terms of being rescued from symbolically suicidal activities. When he insisted that he was ten feet tall and had the biggest of all penises, the therapists insisted that he was really only a young boy, but would some day grow up into a man as big as his father. Mike would react with rage, then appear intensely depressed, and finally begin behaving self-destructively. He destroyed all his art work, defecated on the floor, and attempted to smear the feces over himself. His individual therapist worked diligently with him during this difficult time, giving Mike support in coping with his intense feelings of worthlessness and fear of abandonment. Mike repeatedly referred to Kate (who had been withdrawn from treatment two years previously) and how he had urinated on her, years ago; he insisted that he had destroyed her by this act. He also insisted that he had similarly destroyed Dr. Speers, who now worked with the group only infrequently, but often spoke to the children in the halls of the Clinic. Mike's parents were of little help to him during this period, as they were entertaining conscious fantasies of institutionalizing him, and when angry often told him how bad he was, and how much they hated him.

One gratifying aspect of therapy during the fourth year was the fact that to a large extent the children confined their psychotic behavior to the group sessions, while at school (and to some extent at home) their behavior, though schizoid, was rarely psychotic. The exception was Mike, who was quite difficult at home and repeatedly provoked his mother to hit him and call him worthless. All of the children attended school during this year. Bob at first re-entered the first grade, but after a few weeks moved up to second, where he performed well. He appeared to pay little attention to the teacher and frequently interfered with the other children's activities, but he learned well and performed at grade level. He kept apart from the children on the playground, and instead sought adults to relate to. But he very much wanted to have "friends," and as his mother permitted him more freedom, he was seen further and further away from home while playing. Walter attended a special education class and later a regular first grade. Although he had Mr. Rabbit with him at all times, he was able to ride the bus to school and was virtually never a behavior problem. His achievement tests at the end of the year were at grade level.

Mike repeated the first grade, and although he participated poorly in classroom activities, there was no question that he learned well. He scored above the grade norm on the achievement tests and was promoted to the second grade. Tina attended a special education class and her teacher said that she presented no serious problems. She had to be individually attended to before she could perform, and she preferred to watch the other children rather than participating with them. In situations of stress, she "became" a cat or dog, and behaved in a silly manner, but this delighted the other children, and they did not shame or ridicule her. Carol attended a special education class in which she participated poorly. She gave up her irritating habit of crying all the time, and her speech became more communicative, but her interest in learning remained minimal. She often talked of her little sister and her parents and seemed quite preoccupied with activities at home. Melvin attended a kindergarten for retarded children, and his teacher became very interested in working with him. She assured the mother that he was happiest when with her and wanted to keep Melvin in a small group of children during the summer. The mother was glad to comply, as this provided an extra reason for her to stay home in order to devote more time to her older children when they were out of school.

Darlene attended first grade in her local public school, and although she gave no evidence of any formal learning, she seemed to profit socially from the experience and presented no management problem to the teacher. Shirley was in a special education class and also seemed to profit socially. She was strongly resistant to learning, particularly when this involved following directions: she would point to every word except the right one.

The teachers and social scientists from the group project visited the homes and classrooms of all the children. They reported that every child was obviously different from his contemporaries and stood out in the classroom because of this difference. However, none of the teachers felt that the children were "problems." Walter's teacher was delighted with his progress during the year. She was concerned about his infantile speech, but felt he had learned well and participated in most activities at a near normal level. Bob's teacher was generally satisfied, but expressed concern over his inability to play with the other children. Mike's teacher was disappointed with his performance in school, but delighted (and amazed) at his score on the achievement tests. The observers saw no psychotic behavior at home or in school, but reported schizoid behavior nearly uniformly—Walter was the exception.

At the present time (May, 1964) there is remarkable solidarity in the group. Group interaction is constant and vigorous. Disruptive behavior, though not forbidden, seldom occurs; when it does, it almost always stems from Mike's special distress. The formal teaching program has become fairly sophisticated, with reading, writing, and simple arithmetic. The children enthusiastically approach the craft projects, which have become more and more complex. Attempts are being made to involve the whole group in recreation activities, but the children usually prefer to play in groups of two or three. The swimming parties were held this year without panic and were enjoyed greatly by every child. All the therapists find it easier to give group interpretations, and it is generally agreed that the level of maturity in the group is such that primitive, preverbal feelings and behavior are now the exception, and not the rule.

THIRD AND FOURTH YEARS OF PARENTS' GROUPS

During the third year, group therapy of the parents continued as in the previous two years. The fathers (now with their third therapist) continued to be shy, evasive, and resistant, and avoided feelings as much as possible. Absenteeism was common, and group formation tenuous. The therapist, like previous ones, played a passive "waiting game," but he was pitted against lifelong masters of the passive approach, and tangible progress was very slow. Second-guessing, we later surmised that a more active, supportive, or challenging attitude *might* have stirred things up and led to more active therapy.

The mothers' group (still with RWS as therapist) during the first three months of the third year frequently discussed the possibility of the children's entering school. All the children had gone to kindergarten the year before, and Walter, Tina, and Annaletta would return to kindergarten, while Bob and Mike were to enter a regular first grade. The mothers verbalized concerns about feeling embarrassed if the child should act up in school, but also anticipated hurt and humiliation if the child was unable to remain in school.

The group then began discussing the numerous situations in which they found their pride hurt, and how they reacted to this. The most severe loss of self-esteem occurred when their children failed to behave "normally." When this happened, they found themselves attacking the child and attempting to force him to "act right." We often heard the statement: "I could really love him if he would just act right." The therapist pointed out how each mother also felt that if *she* "acted right" she would be "really loved" by her mother in the past, and in the present by husband and therapist.

In the final three months of the year, the mothers continued to look at their infantile demands and the frustrations and rage they felt when these demands were not fulfilled. Similarly, they became more aware of using the sick child to attain these wishes for themselves (via identification) and also how they used the child as a repository for their own unacceptable impulses. Their relationships with one another in the group, with the therapist, and with their husbands, became more realistic and mature. However, the mothers still suffered feelings of shame and humiliation whenever the child behaved in a bizarre or infantile manner, and they continued to react with coercion or attack.

With this particular point in mind, it was decided to have each mother and child seen simultaneously by an individual therapist, in order to observe, expose, and hopefully modify this pathological interaction. A number of the children were already being seen individually (once or twice weekly) and there was some resistance to putting the new idea into practice. Of those therapists who tried it, none could keep it up for long. In the sessions, the mother nagged, provoked, needled, or verbally attacked the child with intense overt anger and competed strongly with the child for the therapist's attention and "love." The therapist, identifying with the child under attack, found this intolerable, and soon separated mother and child, seeing them individually once or twice a week, or arranging for another therapist for the mother.

This experiment coincided with the beginning of the fourth year of group therapy, at which point, due to staff changes, there was a massive revision of the parent therapy groups.

RWS was forced to give up his mothers' group in order to begin treating a new group of children, and the other group therapists were leaving the area. We decided to combine all the parents (mothers and fathers, "old" and "new") into a single group meeting twice monthly with one of the authors (CL) as therapist.

This change was not much of a novelty for the fathers, but the mothers reacted with rage to the breaking up of their long-standing and exclusive group and the loss of their idealized "mother-therapist." This was worked through not in the combined group, but in individual therapy, and the coincidence of this upheaval with the attempt at mother-child therapy may have accounted for some of the vehemence with which these women competed with their children. Each resorted to her usual characterological method of trying to obtain gratification of her infantile demands, and much that had occurred in previous group therapy now reappeared in the individual sessions. In time this was worked through, however, and each mother made some gains in insight and maturity and in her ability to permit some further separation between herself and the sick child. Mrs. M., however, developed a sexualized dependency transference to her individual therapist, which only increased her hostile, destructive interaction with Mike. It was only after transfer to a woman therapist that her assets as a woman and mother began to emerge in her everyday living and in her interaction with Mike.

The combined parents' group was well attended by the mothers, with a sprinkling of fathers, although sometimes as many as four or five men showed up. Three fathers never attended. Mrs. A. came to one meeting, but was never seen again. Early group formation was tepid and sociable in quality. Personal and conflictual matters were taken up in individual therapy and largely avoided in the group. However, further past and family history was related, and common problems were discussed with interest, such as stingy and depreciatory parental attitudes. The "old" members did most of the talking, and were remarkably polite, for fear (so they said) of frightening the newcomers to the group therapy. However, Mr. W. took to needling his wife, which he never did elsewhere, because he said he knew that the presence of the group would restrain her from retaliatory mayhem. Toward the end of the year Mrs. B. (previously noted for her massive denial of hostility, etc.) complained that there was too much chitchat in the group and no serious discussions. Following this, the members began to develop a tentative common identity as fellow-sufferers, aligned warily against the therapist as an indifferent taskmaster. There was discussion of meeting every week, but the majority wanted to use the free time for relaxation or reading, which, coming from these passive people, may indicate commendable self-assertiveness, as well as resistance.

X · Discussion: Later Phases of Therapy

During the four years of this project, the staff participants repeatedly reviewed the material obtained from the various therapy groups in an effort to formulate the genetics of each child's psychosis and the dynamics of its perpetuation. Since we were dealing with groups rather than individuals, attention was focused on group dynamics. The formulations presented are derived from observation of behavior (including transference manifestations) and from verbalizations within the various groups; they represent ongoing dynamics as well as a reconstruction of past interactions.

THE PARENTS

When the mothers entered group therapy, it was not with insight into their contribution to the child's psychosis, nor with an idea of amending personality defects, but rather in a misguided effort to obtain gratification of previously frustrated narcissistic wishes. From their autobiographies, verbalizations, and transference attitudes, it is evident that their own processes of separation and individuation had been incomplete, and that each had made several attempts to reconstitute a childhood symbiosis. In the group therapy they made yet another attempt to regain symbiosis. The fantasy of the group was clearly one in which personal "perfection" was the chief condition of achieving this goal. To obtain such perfection, socially undesirable and personally unacceptable impulses were rejected. These undesirable impulses, feelings, and thoughts included greed and gluttony; envy and jealously; aggressiveness, hostility, and hate; and all aspects of infantile sexuality. In more general terms, anything designated as "childish" or socially "bad" was included. The mothers saw treatment as a means of eliminating these undesirable qualities and thus attaining an ideal state of perfection with consequent rewards of complete dependency and fulfilment of narcissistic wishes. In their eyes, the sick child represented everything they believed to be reprehensible, and they wished to eliminate the child, or at least eliminate the behavior and substitute perfection for it. In the group therapy sessions, all such unacceptable impulses were attributed to the child, the husband, in-laws, siblings, and ultimately, through role-playing, to other members of the group. The group therapist was related to as though he were an all-knowing, all-giving, all-powerful mother who was demanding perfection from her children. No "bad" feelings, acts, or thoughts were to be shown to this powerful mother, because only a perfect child would be chosen for special rewards. When the rewards failed to materialize, profound rage appeared. In this affect-laden situation, memories of past interactions between mother and infant were expressed and correlated with present interactions.

The basic relationship between mother and child, both in the past and present, was repeatedly shown to be one in which the child failed to live up to the mother's fantasied expectation (which she felt to be a severe criticism of herself), followed by angry attempts on her part to coerce the child to respond as she wished. These coercive activities were initially "loving" acts, but soon developed into tense, angry, rejecting behavior. Innumerable interactions of this type were observed between the mother and child and verbalized by the mothers in the group sessions. Our interpretation of this basic interaction was that the mother saw the child as a means of fulfilling her own needs, with little appreciation that the child had needs of his own. We formulated this in terms of mother's identification with the child, seeing the child as an extension of herself. In either case, "badness" was to be eradicated by "loving" it out of the child, manipulating the child, or rejecting him. Unacceptable behavior or attitudes by any member of the mothers' group, by the husband, in-laws, siblings or friends, was reacted to in a similar manner.

As therapy progressed and the pattern of interaction became evident to the mothers, their relationship with other adults underwent considerable change. This was partly due to insight within the group, but also due to the results of therapy with the fathers, who became increasingly able to tolerate emotional interchange. The mothers and fathers began to express their feelings to each other and thus to communicate their wants, needs, and frustrations. The fathers' pattern of sulking withdrawal (followed by displacement of anger onto the child) markedly decreased, and we noted an increase in their capacity to deal with the mothers. Concomitantly, the fathers were able to identify with the child to a sufficient degree to move in and protect the child from the mother's rage, manipulation, and coercion. However, we were unable to effect what we felt to be an adequate alteration of the basic interaction between mother and child.

Several events forced us to re-evaluate the situation near the end of the third year of therapy: the mothers' group succeeded in displacing and projecting their "badness" onto Mrs. T. who, out of masochistic needs, accepted the role of the "bad sexual child" and defiantly refused to return to the group in spite of repeated interpretations and confrontations by the group therapist. We also realized that the child and mother had unconscious needs to continue their basic interaction (to preserve identity?) and that joint therapy of mother and child might be a more effective means of accomplishing separation-individuation. This process seemed to be well under way in both mother and child, but in certain situations, old symbiotic patterns of interaction persisted. We believed that on-the-spot confrontations could be useful in effecting final separation-individuation. Accordingly, we revised the program to include mother-child sessions with individual therapists in addition to the regular group therapy sessions for the children. The mothers' group was dissolved and replaced with a bi-weekly combined parents' group.

The mothers construed the termination of their group therapy as a rejection. They renewed their efforts to get rid of their fantasied "badness" by projecting and displacing it onto others. The therapists repeatedly interpreted this reaction and although the early mother-child therapy was tense and emotional, the mothers matured noticeably.

The situation in the families at the present time is markedly different from what existed at the onset of therapy. The parents are relating to each other in a co-operative manner whereby feelings can be more openly expressed. The child is less and less an object of scorn, and, in fact, genuine feelings of love have appeared between father and child. In situations of maximal stress (such as the child's school performance) anxiety is evident in the parents, with a tendency to revert to previous patterns. The results obtained so far with the parents is encouraging and suggests that further therapy may permit sufficient maturation to enable them to fulfill more adequately their parental roles. It is our belief that the child cannot separate and individuate without this concurrent maturation in the parents.

THE CHILDREN

The children found the therapy sessions a safe alternative to autism, and ultimately formed a group which served each child as a partner in a therapeutic symbiosis. Our maneuvers in therapy were then directed toward gratifying the real needs of the children in this therapeutic symbiosis, and at the same time encouraging moves toward separation-individuation, and frustrating attempts to reconstitute their familiar magical dyssymbiosis.

We believed that a substantial period in which each child experienced gratification of his real needs (such as being fed when hungry, comforted when hurt or frightened, receiving affection when desired, having potentially destructive impulses prohibited or controlled) would render the group symbiosis not only tolerable, but actually desirable and preferable to the dyssymbiosis. Following this period of repeated need satisfactions, the children responded to impulses to explore the environment, including their own bodies as well as other people. The therapists provided the children with support and encouragement in these endeavors. However, under conditions of increased anxiety, the children quickly reverted to their familiar psychotic patterns of behavior. The therapists frustrated such regression as much as possible and, by providing maximum need satisfaction, encouraged steps forward into separation-individuation.

As a result of these therapeutic attitudes, supports, and interventions, we saw strong group formation and interaction, the development of a group ego with constant boundaries, an increasing degree of impulse control within the group, significant development of affective expression, and ultimately the development of a group identity. Concomitantly, the individual members of the group progressed along similar lines.

Both personal and group identities were quite fragile, however, and therapy was directed towards establishing a constant identity immune to disintegration under ordinary conditions of stress. Anxiety-provoking events which the children distorted, and which represented threats to identity, were ever present and required constant alertness and understanding by the therapists. When such events related to situations at home or to interactions while en route to the sessions, we had great difficulty in understanding and being of assistance to the child. When the event occurred within the group, the therapists' job was somewhat easier. It was imperative to recognize that the reaction of a single child soon affected the entire group, so that group interpretations and interventions were required. For instance, the absence of a child affected group integrity and let to anxiety in the remaining children, each child reacting in his own characteristic way. We initially made simple factual statements to the effect that the child was indeed absent and that we were aware of how this upset the children in the group. We then encouraged verbalization of fantasies about what might have happened to the absent child and ultimately correlated these feelings and fantasies with similar ones which the children had about their own families and themselves. The many other kinds of events which disturbed the sense of identity have been outlined in previous chapters; suffice it to say that we were constantly involved in dealing with this threat. Obviously these interactions strengthened reality testing, promoted ego integration, and advanced separation-individuation. In addition, human relatedness increased, as did the idea of object constancy. As the same time, the children were developing curiosity about the inanimate world and an interest in learning.

In the therapeutic teaching program, we directed our efforts toward furthering the processes mentioned above, as well as using the children's intelligence as another aid to separation-individuation and the establishment of a stable identity. We were also interested in developing techniques which could be used in group teaching of such children. The chief problems were to provide sufficient permissiveness to allow the child to reveal and deal with his current conflicts, and yet to maintain enough structure so that learning could take place. And as we have discussed previously, conflict in an individual child (which if not dealt with may infect the whole group) often results in obsessive fixation on *things,* which blocks learning just as effectively as chaotic behavior.

For a time, the emphasis was chiefly on reality, structure, and learning. When a child became upset, a therapist would supply external control as needed and deal with the child's anxiety while the rest of the group continued their program. Usually brief attention would enable the upset child to rejoin the group. The children were not as a group encouraged to act out fantasies, however. Eventually, rumblings of impulsive aggressive behavior alerted us to the fact that more anxiety existed than could be handled in this casual manner. As soon as external controls were largely removed, a stormy flood of phallic concerns and fantasies were verbalized as well as acted out and became accessible to interpretation. This entailed considerable modification of the educational program, and at times the goals of uncovering therapy seemed inconsistent with the minimal requirements of scholastic discipline. The children continued to behave well at their own schools, but their vehement aggressiveness in the group put great stress on the patience and integrative powers of the teachers and therapists. The general philosophy of expressive therapy called for permissiveness, while instinctive protective reactions cried out for limits and control. No one could predict how far these children might go in attacking one another, and there was no precedent by which to judge how much mayhem we could safely permit. This had not been a problem in the first year because of the children's small size, but three years later it caused genuine concern.

Eventually we realized that one reason the children acted up was to manipulate the adults, *forcing* them to assume the function of an external superego. The adults then withdrew, announcing their refusal to act in this capacity, and telling the children that they would have to exert their own control and terminate their own aggressive behavior. The adults merely controlled certain physical aspects of the situation by removing potential brickbats and furniture when necessary. This permitted the children to "misbehave" as hard as they could, which they seemed to do in a desperate effort to compel adult intervention. But the therapists' relentless determination not to interfere did enable the children to discover that their fiercest destructive, sexual, and aggressive behavior had in fact very little important effect, and demonstrated that their destructive fantasies were seriously limited by simple physical reality, and were in fact impossible to fulfill. It is a sobering but reassuring thing for a seven-year-old to discover that he really is not capable of demolishing another person bare-handed, no matter how badly he wants to. The therapists were also relieved.

The therapy with children and parents continues, and we feel that it is generally effective. However, we are repeatedly impressed with the tenacity of the basic pathological interaction between mother and child. There is definite evidence that mother and child continue to share ego in certain specific areas, clearly related to infantile impulses which the mother has not integrated into her own personality. In addition, the child clings to the vestiges of omnipotence in his ability to "make mother move" in certain stereotyped ways, by provoking irrational behavior. Mother and child may by now have realized that this interaction is futile, but the temptation to provoke it remains strong, even though the need is no longer desperate; it is perhaps a kind of addiction. It is our belief that with continuing therapy, there is a good possibility that the mother will effect the integration of her infantile impulses. Therapy with the child will hopefully promote further separation-individuation and the establishment of a real and rewarding personal identity. At the same time, both mother and child must perhaps undergo a kind of "mourning" to deal with the loss of a familiar (though spurious) part of themselves, so that they may enter the realm of true object relationships, not only within the family, but in the world at large. Here is where the father may play his most important role in the family.

In conclusion, we believe that group therapy is an effective approach to the treatment of psychosis in childhood. The procedure is "out-patient," and keeps the child in the home and the community. We emphasize treatment of the whole family: it is absolutely necessary to involve the mother intensively in therapy and to exert the strongest efforts to involve the father as well, to assist him to give up his psychological absence and to provide the emotional support so urgently needed by his wife and child. The group technique also offers superior training opportunities for students of child psychiatry and for numerous other disciplines interested in working with seriously disturbed children and their families.

XI · Afterthoughts: A Group of
Younger Children

In order to test the efficacy of our techniques and the validity
of some of our formulations, we began a second program of
group therapy in April, 1963. This new group consisted of
six children aged 22 to 33 months. All were psychotic: one
had brain damage as well, one had primary autism, and the
remaining four had symbiotic psychosis. The general plan of
the new program was similar to what we have described in
this monograph, but now with the financial backing of a U. S.
Public Health Service NIMH Grant for a Demonstration Project, No. MH–1206–02.

There have been several definite differences in the group
process during the first year, which may be simply due to
random variability, but which are worth outlining here, in
case they are actually correlated with the younger age of these
children or with some significant difference of parental psychology which led to their much earlier diagnosis and treatment. The chief differences are outlined below:

1) Panic reactions, which did not often occur,
were mild and easily controlled.

2) Group formation was less evident. While this may not be exclusively due to age, it is well known that group formation does not occur to any great extent in normal children as young as these.

3) Wild, destructive, hyperactive behavior was almost entirely absent.

4) Although we took care to avoid having too many toys in the room, these children did not seem to show a tendency to overreact to a multiplicity of objects.

5) Hostile and aggressive behavior toward other children was minimal. Competition over possession of food and toys built up slowly, as the children developed an interest in these things.

6) The children were generally a great deal more passive, their attitudes resembling that of Tina at the start of the original therapy group. A more active approach was required of the therapists.

7) The children were quite unconcerned by the introduction of new members into the group. We took care to add new children only one at a time, and not four at once, as with the original group.

References

Abse, D. W. and J. A. Ewing (1960). Some problems in psychotherapy with schizophrenic patients, *American Journal of Psychotherapy*, **14**:505–519.

Alexander, F. (1954). Some quantitative aspects of psychoanalytic technique, *Journal of the American Psychoanalytic Association*, **2**:685–701.

Bender, L., and A. M. Freedman (1952). A study of the first three years in the maturation of schizophrenic children, *Quarterly Journal of Child Behavior*, **4**:245–272.

Bergman, P., and S. K. Escalona (1949). Unusual sensitivities in very young children, *Psychoanalytic Study of the Child*, **3–4**: 333–352. New York, International Universities Press.

Des Lauriers, A. M. (1962). *The Experience of Reality in Childhood Schizophrenia*, Monograph Series on Schizophrenia, No. 6. New York, International Universities Press.

Eissler, K. R. (1954). Notes upon defects of ego structure in schizophrenia, *International Journal of Psycho-Analysis*, **35**: 141–146.

Federn, P. (1952). *Ego Psychology and the Psychoses*. New York, Basic Books.

Foulkes, S. H., and E. J. Anthony (1957). *Group Psychotherapy: The Psychoanalytic Approach*. Baltimore, Penguin Books.

Hartmann, H. (1953). Contribution to the metapsychology of schizophrenia, *Psychoanalytic Study of the Child*, 8:177–198. New York, International Universities Press.

Jacobsen, E. (1954). Contributions to the metapsychology of psychotic identifications, *Journal of the American Psychoanalytic Association*, 2:239–262.

Kanner, L. (1949). Problems of nosology and psychodynamics of early infantile autism, *American Journal of Orthopsychiatry*, 19:416–426.

Klein, M. (1946). Notes on some schizoid mechanisms, *International Journal of Psycho-Analysis*, 27:99–110.

Knight, R. P. (1953). Borderline states, *Bulletin of the Menninger Clinic*, 17:1–12.

Mahler, M. S., J. R. Ross, Jr., and Z. De Fries (1949). Clinical studies of benign and malignant cases of childhood psychosis (schizophrenia-like), *American Journal of Orthopsychiatry*, 19:295–305.

Mahler, M. S. (1952). On child psychosis and schizophrenia: Autistic and symbiotic infantile psychoses, *Psychoanalytic Study of the Child*, 7:286–305. New York, International Universities Press.

Mahler, M. S. and B. J. Gosliner (1955). On symbiotic child psychosis: genetic, dynamic and restitutive aspects, *Psychoanalytic Study of the Child*, 10:195–212. New York, International Universities Press.

Mahler, M. S., M. Furer, and C. F. Settlage (1959). Severe emotional disturbances in childhood, in S. Arieti (ed.) *American Handbook of Psychiatry*. New York, Basic Books. Vol. 1, pp. 816–839.

Mahler, M. S., and M. Furer (1960). Observations on research regarding the "symbiotic syndrome" of infantile psychosis, *Psychoanalytic Quarterly*, 29:317–327.

Rank, B., and S. Kaplan (1951). A case of pseudo-schizophrenia in a child, *American Journal of Orthopsychiatry*, 21:155–181.

Sperling, M. (1963). Fetishism in children, *Psychoanalytic Quarterly*, 32:374–392.

*9 7 8 0 8 0 7 8 7 9 4 7 4 *